TRACK YOUR PATH BACK TO HEALTH

WHEAT BELLY

JOURNAL

WILLIAM DAVIS, MD

This book is intended as a reference volume only, not as a medical manual.
The information given here is designed to help you make informed decisions about your health.
It is not intended as a substitute for any treatment that may have been prescribed by your doctor.
If you suspect that you have a medical problem, we urge you to seek competent medical help.

Mention of specific companies, organizations, or authorities in this book does not imply endorsement
by the author or publisher, nor does mention of specific companies, organizations, or authorities
imply that they endorse this book, its author, or the publisher.

Internet addresses and telephone numbers given in this book
were accurate at the time it went to press.

© 2013 by William Davis, MD

Printed in the United States of America

Rodale Inc. makes every effort to use acid-free, recycled paper.

ISBN 978–1–62336–070–2 paperback

Distributed to the trade by Macmillan

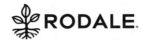

We inspire and enable people to improve their lives and the world around them.
rodalebooks.com

INTRODUCTION

Numerous studies have proven that keeping a food journal doubles your weight loss and sets you on the path to long-term health. So what better way to help you eliminate your wheat belly than by providing you with the single most effective weight-loss tool available?

This journal was specifically designed to accompany *Wheat Belly* and help you purge the single greatest-known supercarbohydrate from your body: wheat. By allowing you to track your daily vitals, what you eat, and how you feel as you eliminate wheat from your diet, this book will serve as a written account that raises your self-awareness, motivates you to maintain your new diet plan, and helps you identify just how wheat was affecting your life. By removing wheat from your meals, you'll not only transition into a life free of belly fat, digestive problems, allergies, and cravings, but also improve the following conditions:

- Obesity
- Inflammation
- Heart disease
- Diabetes

- Arthritis
- Mental fatigue
- Skin problems

Gone are the days of succumbing to your health issues. Are you ready to find the thinner, more energetic, clearer-thinking you? Are you ready to regain control of your weight, and your life? Turn the page to learn how to banish your wheat belly and your wheat-dependent life for good!

Brace Yourself for Health

While eliminating wheat from your diet may be inconvenient at first, it is certainly not unhealthy. For years you've been told "healthy whole grains" are an integral component of a well-balanced diet. But this simply isn't true. The majority of people who eliminate wheat from their diets experience:

- Flatter tummy
- Lower triglycerides
- Higher HDL ("good") cholesterol
- Normal blood sugar
- Normal blood pressure
- Normal bowel function

You can also expect to have more energy, better sleep, and weight loss. (Those on a wheat-free diet naturally consume 350 to 400 fewer calories per day.)

While removing wheat is the first step in achieving ideal health, it's essential to be mindful of the foods you are choosing to replace the lost wheat calories. Replacing your wheat calories with highly processed, herbicide-covered, genetically modified, ready-to-eat, high-fructose corn syrup–filled, or just-add-water food products will not move you closer to your goal. Choose whole foods such as vegetables, raw nuts, and protein, which will increase your fiber or protein intake.

Schedule Your Radical Wheat-Ectomy

It may be daunting to think about removing wheat from your diet completely. After all, it's likely a large component of your daily intake. Thankfully, eliminating all wheat from your diet is not as painful as you may first believe.

The most effective and, ultimately, the easiest way to eliminate wheat is to do it abruptly and completely. The insulin-glucose roller coaster caused by wheat, along with the addictive effects of exorphins, the opiate derived from the digestion of wheat proteins, makes it difficult for some people to reduce wheat gradually. Abrupt and complete elimination of wheat will, in the susceptible, trigger the withdrawal phenomenon. But getting through the withdrawal that accompanies abrupt cessation may be easier than the gnawing fluctuations of cravings that usually accompany just cutting back. Nonetheless, some people are more comfortable with gradual reduction. Either way, the end result is the same: Removing wheat will set you free.

To begin, eliminate all wheat-based products: breads, breakfast cereals, noodles, pasta, bagels, muffins, pancakes, waffles, doughnuts, pretzels, crackers, and oat products. Although these foods may have been common in your previous diet, their removal is essential for a successful wheat-free lifestyle.

WHEAT WITHDRAWAL TIPS

Your first few wheat-free days can bring on unpleasant withdrawal symptoms. These strategies can help make your transition a bit more tolerable:

- Drink lots of water throughout the day.
- Begin your journey during a low-stress period like a slow work week.
- Take a probiotic (e.g., 50 billion CFUs or greater per day) to accelerate the recovery of normal bowel flora and minimize gas, cramps, and constipation.
- Take a vitamin D supplement to make you feel clearer and stronger. Most adults require 6,000 units per day in gelcap form.

Other Carbohydrates

So what's next after you've removed the wheat from your diet? While you've eliminated the biggest problem in your diet, other carbohydrates can be culprits as well.

Excessive carbohydrate consumption can expose you to steep fluctuations of blood sugar, increasingly severe resistance to insulin, growth of belly (visceral) fat, and inflammatory responses. So reducing your overall carbohydrate intake is extremely beneficial.

If you want to maximize the benefits of your new wheat-free lifestyle, or if substantial weight loss is among your health goals, then you should also consider reducing or eliminating the following foods:

- **Cornstarch and cornmeal**—Cornmeal products such as tacos, tortillas, corn chips, and corn breads, breakfast cereals, and sauces and gravies thickened with cornstarch.

- **Snack foods**—Potato chips, rice cakes, popcorn. These foods, like foods made of cornstarch, send blood sugar straight up to the stratosphere.

- **Desserts**—Pies, cakes, cupcakes, ice cream, sherbet, and other sugary desserts all pack too much sugar.

- **Potatoes**—White, red, and sweet potatoes and yams generate adverse blood sugar effects.

- **Gluten-free foods**—Because the cornstarch, rice starch, potato starch, and tapioca starch used in place of wheat gluten cause extravagant rises in blood sugar, they should be avoided.

- **Fruit juices, soft drinks**—While they contain healthy components such as flavonoids and vitamin C, even the "natural" fruit juices are not good for you. Small servings of 2 to 4 ounces are generally fine, but these drinks are high in sugar, so more than a few ounces will raise your blood sugar. Carbonated soft drinks are incredibly unhealthy, mostly due to added sugars, high-fructose corn syrup, colorings, and the extreme acid challenge from the carbonation.

- **Dried fruit**—Dried cranberries, raisins, figs, dates, apricots.

While there is no need to restrict fats when switching to a wheat-free diet, certain fats and fatty foods should be avoided. These include hydrogenated (trans) fats in processed foods, fried oils that contain excessive by-products of oxidation and advanced glycation end-product (AGE) formation, and cured meats (sodium nitrite and AGEs).

SUGAR SUBSTITUTES

Craving something sweet, but don't want to deal with the physiological consequences of sugar? Try these sugar substitutes:

Stevia: While not interchangeable with sugar, preparation instructions usually provide advice on what quantity of stevia matches the sweetness of sugar.

Xylitol: Xylitol yields two-thirds of the calories of table sugar and can be used interchangeably with sugar in recipes—and has the least effect on baking characteristics.

Erythritol: Erythritol has a unique "cooling" sensation, like peppermint, but does not hold up in baking as well as other sweeteners.

Sucralose: Sucralose, aka Splenda, is very baking-compatible. Although there have been negative reports on sucralose, there is no formal evidence of these side effects.

Wheat Belly Foods (What Can I Eat?)

This is the very same diet I advise for patients in my office that achieves spectacular reductions in small LDL particles (the number-one cause of heart disease in the United States) and unravels diabetic and prediabetic tendencies. The biggest step is the elimination of wheat and then carbohydrates. But what's left after you've eliminated wheat and the carbohydrates listed on pages 8–9 from your diet? There are several basic principles that will serve you well in your wheat-free campaign.

The Wheat Belly Nutritional Approach for Optimal Health

Here's a handy summary of the foods you can enjoy with abandon, those you should eat in limited quantities, and those that should only rarely be a part of your diet.

EAT ALL YOU WANT

Vegetables, except potatoes and corn (fresh or frozen, never canned)

Raw nuts and seeds: raw almonds, walnuts, pecans, hazelnuts, pistachios,

Brazil nuts, cashews, dry-roasted peanuts (not roasted in oil), ground flaxseed, chia seeds, pumpkin seeds, and sunflower seeds

Healthy oils (unheated): olive, flaxseed, coconut, avocado, walnut

Meats: red meats, pork, fish, chicken, turkey, eggs (Consider free-range, grass-fed, and/or organic sources.)

Teas, coffee, water, unsweetened almond milk, coconut milk, or coconut water

Cheeses: real cultured cheeses only (not Velveeta or single-slice processed cheese)

Avocado or guacamole; hummus; unsweetened condiments, e.g., may-onnaise, mustard, oil-based salad dressings; ketchup without high-fructose corn syrup; pesto, tapenades; olives, coconut, cocoa (unsweetened), or cacao

EAT IN LIMITED QUANTITIES

Fruit: No more than 2 servings a day (1 serving is a level handful), preferably in this order (best first): berries of all varieties, citrus, apples, nectarines, peaches, melons. See the Fruit Scale on the next page.

Minimize bananas, pineapples, mangoes, and grapes.

Fruit juices: Only 100-percent juice and in minimal quantities (no more than 2 to 4 ounces)

Nonwheat, nongluten grains—Stick to a ½-cup serving or less.

Whole corn (not to be confused with cornmeal or cornstarch, which should be avoided)

Noncheese dairy products: No more than 1 serving per day of milk, cottage cheese, or yogurt

Legumes and beans (stick to a ½-cup serving or less): peas, sweet potatoes and yams, rice (white and brown), soy

Dark chocolates, 70 to 85 percent cocoa or greater (no more than 40 grams)

Sugar-free foods—Preferably stevia-containing

Soy products

EAT RARELY OR NEVER

Fried foods

Fast foods

Unhealthy oils—(especially corn, sunflower, safflower, grapeseed, cottonseed, soybean)

Hydrogenated "trans" fats

Dried fruit

Cured meats: hot dogs, sausages, bacon, bologna, pepperoni

High-fructose corn syrup–containing foods, honey, agave syrup, sucrose (table sugar)

Sugary snacks, condiments, and sweeteners

Processed rice, rice flour, or potato products: rice crackers, rice cereals, pretzels, white breads, breakfast cereals, potato chips

Fat-free or low-fat salad dressings

"Gluten-free" foods—specifically those made with cornstarch, rice starch, potato starch, or tapioca starch

QUICK TIPS:

For healthy breakfast choices, consider ground flaxseed as a hot cereal (e.g., with soy milk, milk, or unsweetened almond milk; blueberries, strawberries, etc.). Also consider having "dinner for breakfast"—eating salads, cheese, chicken, and other "dinner" foods for breakfast.

Add 1 teaspoon or more of taste-compatible healthy oil to every meal. For example, mix 1 tablespoon of flaxseed oil into ground flaxseed hot cereal. Or add 2 tablespoons of olive oil to eggs after scrambling. Adding oils will blunt your appetite.

If you suspect you have a wheat "addiction," use the first week to add healthy oils to every meal and reduce the amount of wheat by half. In the second week, aim for elimination of wheat while maintaining the oils.

Reach for raw nuts first as a convenient snack.

The Wheat Belly Fruit Scale

Choosing the most nutritious fruits, meaning the richest in health-promoting flavonoids/antioxidants, while also selecting ones that have the lowest sugar content, is key. Portion control is also crucial. For most fruit, staying at ½ cup per serving will keep your sugar intake at a healthy level. Here's a quick guide to fruit from the best on down to the not so good:

BERRIES

Berries have the greatest amounts of healthy flavonoids. Berries pack the greatest nutrient content with the least sugar. Wonderful berries include:

- Acai
- Bearberries
- Bilberries
- Blackberries
- Blueberries
- Cherries
- Chokeberries
- Cranberries
- Goji berries
- Gooseberries
- Huckleberries
- Kiwifruit ("kiwi")
- Pomegranate (berrylike in its nutritional composition)
- Raspberries
- Strawberries
- Wolfberries

CITRUS

Rich in vitamin C and flavonoids, citrus fruits provide unique health effects. The key is serving size: Keep it small. In the list below, kumquats have the lowest net carbs, while tangerines and clementines have the highest.

- Clementines
- Grapefruit
- Kumquats
- Lemons
- Limes
- Oranges
- Pomelo
- Tangerines

COMMON FRUIT

These popular fruits are listed because they have become American dietary staples. Note that grapes and plums contain higher net carbohydrates than the fruit listed below, so limit your portion sizes.

- Apples
- Apricots
- Nectarines
- Peaches
- Pears

MELONS

Melons have carbohydrate content similar to other fruit, generally 6 to 7 grams per ½-cup serving. They are generally consumed in far greater quantities, however, so make sure to measure what you're going to eat.

- Cantaloupe
- Casaba
- Crenshaw
- Honeydew
- Muskmelon
- Watermelon

TROPICAL FRUIT

Tropical fruits provide the most potential for overexposure to sugars. Even a ½-cup serving may challenge your sugar tolerance. Bananas enjoy an undeserved place as the most popular fruit in the world, as they contain too much sugar. Pineapple and mango are next in line, each with 12.5 grams net carbs per ½ cup. Tropical fruits are therefore best consumed in the smallest quantities—for example, ¼ cup or half of a banana at a time.

A Wheat Belly Shopping List

Now that you've tossed out all of the wheat-based products listed on page 6, it's time to restock your kitchen shelves with necessities that will help you achieve your goal of a wheat-free diet. Certain foods are essential cornerstones in a nutritious, wheat-free life. We use these foods as basic ingredients in one-of-a-kind recipes that make the transition into a wheat-free lifestyle convenient and painless.

Be sure to take advantage of local farmers' markets, butchers, and grocers, because these vendors can be trusted to be free of grain traces that many processed foods contain. By visiting local markets, you create a solid, single-ingredient foundation for your kitchen that will make living a wheat-free lifestyle easier and more enjoyable.

Unfortunately, not all food is single-ingredient food that can be purchased at a nearby outdoor market. This is where reading labels becomes important. Some products to be avoided are clearly marked with words like "wheat," "gluten," or other buzzwords for wheat. Avoiding blatantly wheat-labeled products is a start, but complications arise when trying to determine what does or does not contain wheat. Some dietary guesswork will be necessary, and everyone is mistakenly exposed to wheat at some point. When you find yourself questioning wheat's presence in a particular product, it is helpful to search the manufacturer's website or even personally contact the manufacturer. If the information you receive is still unclear, as in "it's a wheat- and gluten-free product but is not produced in a gluten-free facility," consuming the product should not be risky, although those who are very sensitive should consider avoiding the product.

When shopping for your new wheat-free lifestyle, be sure to take cost into account. While gluten-free foods are generally more costly because they do not receive the government subsidies that wheat receives, there are ways of finding foods that are both affordable and wheat free. Shopping around and researching store prices is absolutely crucial, because the prices of many gluten-free foods have vary greatly. Ground almonds, for example, can be purchased anywhere from $3 per pound to $18.99 per pound. This dramatic difference in price may be due to a variance in flour quality, but many delicious, wheat-free products can be made from the inexpensive $3 flour.

It is important to note that some wheat-free staples like flaxseed, chia, and nut meals should be consumed within 4 weeks to avoid oxidation of the oils, especially if they are preground. Once ground, airtight containers in the refrigerator or freezer will help to keep your gluten-free snacks fresher for a longer time.

Almond meal, almond flour. Almond meal ground from whole almonds and almond flour ground from blanched almonds are cornerstones of wheat flour replacements. They slip seamlessly into all of our baked recipes where nut meal or flour is needed. Those who are skeptical or unfamiliar with using almonds this way will be pleasantly surprised at their light and non-nutty taste when used in our recipes. When you are striving for a very light texture, for example when baking a layer cake, be sure to have some almond flour in your kitchen. Almond meal, which is coarser, less costly, and readily available, is a better alternative for everyday uses than almond flour.

Almond milk, unsweetened. Almond milk is versatile, useful for drinking, baking, and as the milk in grainless "granolas." Almond milk, thinner than cow's milk, is created by first crushing almonds and then collecting the leftover liquid. It is possible to make your own by pureeing almonds and straining the liquid left over through a material like cheesecloth. After, dilute the milk with water to achieve the thickness you want. The leftover pulp can be used later for baking. Like other wheat-free products, skip the sweetened variety and instead opt to control the amount of sweetness yourself through sweeteners.

Baking powder. Although wheat-free flours and meals do not rise as much as their wheat counterparts do, many use baking powder to make rising easier. There are two options when searching for baking powder. First, you can keep an eye out for wheat-free and aluminum-free preparations. Or you can create your own baking powder by mixing cream of tartar and baking soda, 2:1. Be sure to store your baking powder in a sealed, airtight container.

Cauliflower. When recipes call for mashed potations, rice, or stuffing, you can substitute cauliflower for a fresh, wheat-free alternative.

Cheeses. Be sure to keep several cheeses on hand, especially Parmesan, mozzarella, and ricotta. To add a pinch of zest to your Italian dishes, grated Romano and Parmesan are perfect. When experimenting with flatbread recipes made with nut meals and flour, add cheese ground down to a granular consistency. Because nut meal can sometimes have a crumbly texture, melted cheese is an excellent way to keep your dish delicious and in one piece.

Chia seeds. Although not necessarily crucial, chia seeds make for a very compelling addition to a recipe. Chia lovers often grind this interesting seed to use as another baking flour or even add it to their smoothies. Chia seeds strangely expand upon their introduction into water, which makes them helpful when creating mousses and puddings.

Chocolate. Most people love the allure of a rich, chocolate taste in their recipes. This is why 100 percent or unsweetened chocolate, i.e., cacao with cacao butter but no sugar, is very useful in a wheat-free diet. In addition, you can determine just how much sweetness you want in your recipe by adding your own sweetener to the melted chocolate, whereas with ready-made chocolate you cannot. Interestingly, the longer you are wheat free, the less you will require sweetener. Ghirardelli and Baker's are two of the most popular unsweetened chocolates commonly used.

Chocolate chips. To limit sugar content, skip milk chocolate and instead purchase semisweet, dark, or 60 percent cacao chocolate chips. The darkest chocolate chips will typically contain approximately 8 grams "net" carbohydrates (total carbohydrates minus fiber) per 15-gram serving. However, for those of you who are extremely gluten sensitive, be sure to look for wheat-free chips.

Cocoa powder, unsweetened. Good examples of unsweetened powder brands are Ghirardelli, Scharffen Berger, Hershey, and Trader Joe's. Using cocoa powder is perfect for the health-conscious consumer because unlike ready-made chocolate, unsweetened powders allow you to control sweetness levels.

Coconut, shredded and unsweetened; coconut flakes. If you are looking to add flavor and texture to your baked goods, unsweetened coconut is ideal. In addition, coconut is rich in potassium and fiber.

Coconut flour. No wheat-free kitchen is complete without coconut flour, which combines very nicely with nut meals and flours to make baked goods finer and less crumbly. Coconut flour is made by grinding dried coconut meat and should be stored in an airtight container to reduce water absorbency.

Coconut milk. Many varieties of coconut milk are available for your new wheat-free recipes. Thick varieties are perfect when recipes require sour cream or thickeners and are generally sold in cans. Thinner coconut milk, found in cartons, is useful as a go-to substitute for milk whether for your cereal or for your baking needs. Carton versions are a good choice for anyone who wishes to avoid bisphenol A in cans, but if your recipe needs thickening, just add shredded or flaked coconut in your food processor to obtain the correct consistency.

In addition, if you grind down coconut meat with water and strain the coarse remains, you can make any consistency of coconut milk. Currently, only Native Forest canned coconut milk is declared as organic and BPA free.

Cream of tartar. For stiffening egg whites in baking recipes to create a lighter and fluffier result, cream of tartar (aka potassium bitartrate) is ideal. You should use ¼ teaspoon per two egg whites, in bread recipes where "rise" is desired. To minimize aluminum present in most commercial baking powders, just combine cream of tartar 2:1 with baking soda.

Dried fruit. Be sure to purchase unsweetened, dried apricots, cranberries, currants, blueberries, strawberries, and dates to avoid unhealthy sugar loads common in their sweetened counterparts.

Eggs. Because eggs are a major staple in a wheat-free diet, be sure to stock up. Organic eggs from free-range chickens are best and often appear green, blue, or brown with rich yellow yolks. However, organic eggs tend to be pricier than regular eggs, so use your budgetary discretion when grocery shopping.

Extracts. When your baked goods need more flavor, natural almond, coconut, vanilla, and peppermint extracts are great additions.

Flaxseeds. For your wheat-free cereals and baked goods, flaxseeds are crucial because they are rich in both fiber, which increases bowel regularity, and linolenic acid. Skip brown flaxseeds and choose golden flaxseeds, which can be purchased either preground or whole to grind yourself to make baking as smooth as possible.

Ground nut meals. Ground almond, pecan, walnut, and hazelnut meals are very useful in the wheat-free lifestyle, especially as wheat flour replacements.

Guar gum. For delicate wheat-free baked goods that need stiffening, turn to guar gum as an effective thickener. For instance, use ½ teaspoon of guar gum per cup of almond meal recipe or add it in your homemade ice cream and dessert recipes.

Nut and seed butters. Almond butter, peanut butter, and sunflower seed butter can be purchased as preground butters, or you can make your own by grinding the whole nuts in your food processor.

Nuts. Chopped walnuts and pecans are good additions when baking, and raw nuts like almonds, pecans, walnuts, pistachios, hazelnuts, macadamias, and Brazil nuts are also a must in your wheat-free kitchen.

Oils. When shopping, be sure to look for extra-virgin, extra-light olive, coconut, avocado, flaxseed, and walnut oils, plus organic butter.

Seeds. Stock up on raw sunflower, pumpkin, sesame, and chia seeds that are useful ground into flours and used in baking. Other uses for raw seeds such as these include their addition whole in nongrain "granola," or included for more texture in cookies and bars.

Shirataki noodles. An ideal replacement for unhealthy noodles and pastas is shirataki noodles, made from the konjac root, which pack almost no carbohydrates. Shirataki noodles are best in Asian recipes, although they can be used in any pasta recipe. When shopping for shirataki noodles, head straight for the refrigerator section. They are usually packaged in single-serve, liquid-filled bags. Don't worry about the slight fishy odor upon opening the package and rinse the noodles before boiling.

Sweeteners. When searching for sweeteners, rely on liquid stevia, powdered stevia (preferably with inulin, not maltodextrin), powdered erythritol, Truvia, and xylitol. Splenda is widely available, although some people feel sensitive about using this type of sweetener.

Xanthan gum. For creating stronger and more cohesive dough, xanthan gum works well as a thickener. It works best when you use ½ teaspoon per cup of nut/seed meal. Xanthan gum is also useful for making ice cream or iced coconut desserts.

Keeping a variety of vinegars (white, rice, red wine, balsamic—beware the sugar—and infused); several dried herbs and spices; fresh herbs like basil, oregano, and cilantro; fresh garlic and shallots; and different types of mushrooms (cremini, shiitake, portobello) are all very helpful when stocking a wheat-free kitchen.

You should try to purchase meats like beef, turkey, chicken, and pork from organic, trusted sources that are free range, pasture fed, and hormone free. Similarly, avoid purchasing farmed fish and opt for wild-caught, since farmed fish often contain altered fat levels (more omega-6).

If you consume dairy products like cheese, sour cream, butter, yogurt, and milk, try to select organic options to minimize the presence of growth hormones. Once again, organic can be pricey, so choose organic as much as your budget permits.

Kitchen Tools

The tools you already have in your kitchen should not need to change much to adapt to your wheat-free lifestyle. Just think about replacing any tools with porous surfaces like wooden spoons and cutting boards. Simply wash any tools that have previously been used to make anything with wheat.

Be sure to extensively clean pots, dishes, pans, utensils, and appliances like blenders if you are highly gluten sensitive. Be careful if others in your household are not wheat free. In this case, purchasing a second set of utensils and plates may be a good idea. Be wary of any tool with multiple surfaces, cracks, or joints, because wheat crumbs can accumulate there, out of sight. If there are wheat eaters in your household, be sure to purchase a set of porous wooden spoons, cutting board, and other utensils for your own use and explain to others that your utensils are for your use only. Perhaps even purchase tools in a different color to make this transition as smooth as possible.

A few small adjustments may be required for everyone following a wheat-free lifestyle.

Muffin pan. If you do not already have one, consider purchasing a pan with small to medium-size cups, rather than with large or superlarge cups. With large cups, it is often difficult to get the interior of nut- or seed-based meals/flours to bake with the exterior, but using small cups solves this problem. If you want to use a pan with large cups, either bake longer at a lower temperature or use less batter to make a shorter muffin.

Muffin cups. If you decide to use muffin cups, cleaning pans will become much faster and easier. Opt for reusable silicone muffin cups as a cost-effective and environmentally sound option.

Electric hand mixer. If you do not already have an electric hand mixer, consider purchasing one to use during egg preparation. Whipping egg whites first (and using cream of tartar) helps to increase the lightness of baked goods to help them rise more easily.

Food chopper/food processor. When it comes to chopping nuts and seeds into meals and flours and pureeing fruits to use in sweeteners, a food processor is an enormous help. Unfortunately, cleaning a food processor can become a tedious process. Because of this, the KitchenAid food chopper ($40) is an asset to any kitchen, with its strong motor that is not stalled by nuts, seeds, or veggies, while also making cleanup very easy.

Ice cream maker. If you have a sweet tooth but want to avoid the sugary grocery store brands, consider purchasing an ice cream maker. Unless you enjoy cranking a hand-operated maker for hours, spring for an electric ice cream maker. Another perk of owning your own ice cream maker is the ability to experiment with new flavors—try coconut milk–based ice "creams."

Waffle maker. There's no need to give up waffles now that you're wheat free! Make wheat-free waffles with any typical waffle maker.

Whoopie pans. Although you won't be using whoopie pans to make whoopie pies, the extra-shallow cups on whoopie pans are great for wheat-free dough that lacks sturdiness. More uniform heat is delivered to the dough, making small biscuits and breads easier to bake.

Wooden picks. When it comes to wheat-free baking, wooden picks are a must to ensure your baked goods are completely done. Wheat-free products often have trouble baking on the inside, because they are denser than wheat products. Wooden picks allow you to test whether the inside is dry. If the pick is dry upon pulling it out of the product, your baked good is likely baked evenly on the inside. If batter coats the pick, bake the product for a few extra minutes and test again.

Getting Started: A Week of a Wheat-Free Life

Because wheat has become an integral ingredient in our meals—especially breakfast—you may have a hard time envisioning what your meals will look like without it.

Here is a sample of what a weeklong wheat-free diet looks like. Once wheat is eliminated and an otherwise thoughtful approach to diet is followed—i.e., replacing processed food with nutrient-rich food—there is no need to count calories.

The only common diet variable in this approach is carbohydrate content. Most people do best by maintaining a daily carbohydrate intake of approximately 50 and occasionally as high as 100 grams. If you're trying to reverse prediabetes or diabetes, though, you may need to adhere to an even stricter carbohydrate limit of less than 30 grams per day. And if you exercise for prolonged periods, you will likely need to increase your carbohydrate intake during exercise.

Note that serving sizes specified are therefore just suggestions, not restrictions. Recipes in italics can be found in the *Wheat Belly Cookbook*, and recipes in bold can be found in *Wheat Belly*.

DAY 1

BREAKFAST

Crepes with Ricotta and Strawberries (page 100)

LUNCH

Large tomato stuffed with tuna or crabmeat salad

Selection of mixed olives, cheeses, pickled vegetables

DINNER

Beef Burgundy with Fettuccine (page 167)

Mixed green salad (or mixed red and green leaf lettuce) with radicchio, chopped cucumber, sliced radishes, *Vinaigrette Dressing* (page 265)

Lemon Cheesecake Cupcakes (page 260)

DAY 2

BREAKFAST

Granola (page 242)

Apple Walnut "Bread" spread with natural peanut butter, almond butter, cashew butter, or sunflower seed butter (page 257)

LUNCH

Baked portobello mushroom stuffed with crabmeat and goat cheese

DINNER

Grilled tilapia with paprika, thyme, cumin, garlic powder, salt, and pepper

Roasted asparagus and bell peppers with 1 tablespoon of extra-virgin olive oil, salt, and pepper

Chocolate Peanut Butter Fudge (page 264)

DAY 3

BREAKFAST

Eggs scrambled with 2 tablespoons of extra-virgin olive oil, sun-dried tomatoes, and freshly shaved Parmesan

Handful of raw almonds, walnuts, pecans, or pistachios

LUNCH

Greek salad with black or kalamata olives, chopped cucumber, tomato wedges, cubed feta cheese, and extra-virgin olive oil with fresh lemon juice or **Vinaigrette Dressing** (page 265)

DINNER

Baked chicken seasoned with thyme and rosemary

Asparagus with Roasted Garlic and Olive Oil (page 255)

Mocha Walnut Brownies (page 270)

DAY 4

BREAKFAST

Grilled Cheese Breakfast Bake (page 102)

LUNCH

Avocado stuffed with egg salad

Granola (page 242)

DINNER

Parmesan-Breaded Pork Chops with Balsamic-Roasted Vegetables (page 253)

Strawberry Shortcakes (page 251)

DAY 5

BREAKFAST

Berry Coconut Smoothie (page 241)

Handful of raw almonds, walnuts, pecans, or pistachios

LUNCH

Turkey Brie Sandwich (page 119)

Cream of Tomato Soup (page 155)

DINNER

Shirataki Noodle Stir-Fry (page 250)

Ginger Spice Cookies (page 261)

DAY 6

BREAKFAST

Hot Coconut Flaxseed Cereal (page 243)

LUNCH

Mixed green salad (or mixed red and green leaf lettuce) with roasted chicken, hard-boiled eggs, tomatoes, avocado, and cheese with fresh lime juice or *Vinaigrette Dressing* (page 265)

DINNER

Omelet with spinach, sun-dried tomatoes, goat cheese, and chopped vegetables

Apple Walnut "Bread" with cream cheese or pumpkin butter (page 257)

DAY 7

BREAKFAST

Caprese salad (sliced tomato, sliced mozzarella, basil leaves, extra-virgin olive oil)

LUNCH

Pesto Chicken Pizza (page 134)

Ginger Spice Cookies (page 261)

DINNER

Three-Cheese Eggplant Bake (page 256)

Classic Cheesecake with Wheatless Crust (page 263)

This 7-day menu illustrates the variety possible in adapting standard recipes into those that are healthy and wheat free. And you can easily use simple dishes that require little advance planning. Preparing meals without wheat is really easier than you may think. With little more effort than it takes to iron a shirt, you can prepare several meals a day that center on nutritious food, provide the variety necessary for true health, and are free of wheat.

BETWEEN MEALS

On the Wheat Belly diet plan, you may find yourself wanting an occasional snack. Healthy snack choices include:

Raw nuts

Cheese

Dark chocolates—The best choices contain 85 percent or more cacao.

Low-carb crackers—These should be only an occasional indulgence.

Pair with tasty dips like hummus, guacamole, cucumber dip, or salsa.

Vegetable dips

There is truly an incredible range and variety of foods to choose from to fill your wheat gap. It may require you to venture outside your usual shopping and cooking habits, but you will find a variety of flavors to enjoy.

No Going Back—Maintaining Your Wheat-Free Life

Now that you've banished wheat from your diet, your pants are fitting a little better. You have more energy during the day because you're getting a better night's sleep. And that brain fog you had? Gone! You're loving your new lease on life, and you never want to go back to wheat. So how can you maintain your new wheat-free life? Here are a few tips to successfully stay on track.

- **The outer circle.** Once you begin the wheat-free diet plan, you'll find that you spend more time in the produce aisle, farmers' market, or vegetable stand, as well as the butcher shop and dairy aisle. Make sure those middle aisles of your supermarket remain a distant memory.

- **Keep your shopping list close by.** Refer to your shopping list provided in Appendix A of *Wheat Belly*. Whether shopping for groceries or eating out with your family, this list may help you steer clear of foods containing wheat.

- **The removal factor.** Eating outside the home can be a land mine of wheat temptation: cornstarch, sugar, high-fructose corn syrup, and other unhealthy ingredients will be thrust upon you at every turn. If a waiter brings a basket of warm, fragrant rolls to your table, you've just got to turn them away. Remove them from your sight.

- **Keep it simple.** When eating out, baked salmon with a ginger sauce or grilled steak with steamed vegetables is a safe bet. But a multi-ingredient dish has more potential for unwanted ingredients. In the end, eating out of the home presents hazards that may be minimized by selecting simple, straight-forward meals. Whenever possible, eat food so you can be certain of what is contained in your meal.

- **Learn the wheat hiding places.** Numerous items contain hidden wheat ingredients that you'd never expect. Keep an eye out for these possible culprits:
  - Salad dressings—Unless they are labeled as gluten-free. Substitute simple oil and vinegar or a tart lime or lemon juice.
  - Gluten-free pasta—Make sure the utensils used to cook the noodles weren't also used for cooking wheat products.
  - Soy sauce—This popular Asian side almost always contains wheat. Just say no or use a gluten-free soy sauce.

REPLACEMENT INGREDIENTS
FOR OTHER FOOD SENSITIVITIES

Wheat isn't the only substance that may cause adverse effects. The table below outlines substitutions that fit perfectly into a wheat-free lifestyle.

IF YOU ARE SENSITIVE TO:	CONSIDER REPLACING WITH:
Almonds	Chia seed meal, garbanzo bean (chickpea) flour, pecan meal, pumpkin seed meal, sesame seed meal, sunflower seed meal, walnut meal
Butter	Oils: Avocado, coconut, extra-light olive, and walnut
Eggs	Applesauce, chia seeds, coconut milk (canned variety), Greek yogurt (unsweetened), ground flaxseed, pumpkin puree, tofu (from non-GMO soy)
Milk	Almond milk, coconut milk (carton variety), hemp milk, soy milk (from non-GMO soy)
Nuts	Chia seeds (whole, flour), garbanzo bean (chickpea) flour, pumpkin seeds (meal, butter), sesame seeds (whole, flour), sunflower seeds (meal, butter)
Peanut butter	Almond, hazelnut, and sunflower seed butter
Sour cream	Coconut milk (canned variety)

How to Use This Journal

On the following pages you'll find journal logs to help you track the first 12 weeks of your new wheat-free life. Whether you choose to eliminate wheat gradually or immediately, you will find that the logs keep you headed in the right direction.

This journal is your easy, handy tool designed to help you monitor your weight, blood pressure, and blood sugar level daily, which can be an incredible motivator to stay committed to your wheat-free life. You'll be amazed at all you have accomplished when you look back to the beginning of your journey.

Keeping a record of your daily meals is especially helpful if you're struggling to stay on track. Remember: There's no need to count calories. And make sure you note your favorite recipes and snacks! It can be a great guide for the future.

Other markers included in the logs (sleep quality, wheat temptation, and overall mood) are additional ways to measure your progress. Once you eliminate your wheat intake, these markers should improve greatly.

The Additional Comments/Progress section is dedicated to any other notes or accomplishments you want to record. Did you start this wheat-free diet hoping to improve a specific condition? Are your pants noticeably looser today? Use this section to tailor the journal to fit your specific needs. And take note of the weekly testimonials and tips included in this section from Wheat Belly Blog readers who have already made the transition. Use them as a tool to keep you on track in the days ahead.

SAMPLE JOURNAL PAGES

WEEK 1—DAY 1

DATE: 10/1	WEIGHT: 205
BLOOD PRESSURE: 140/85	BLOOD SUGAR A.M./P.M.: 130/109

BREAKFAST:

Granola, Apple Walnut "Bread"

SNACK 1:

Handful of raw almonds

LUNCH:

Grilled Chicken Caesar Salad, ½ cup blueberries

SNACK 2:

Sliced bell peppers and hummus

DINNER:

Pecan-Encrusted Chicken with Tapenade, Asparagus
with Roasted Garlic and Olive Oil

SNACK 3:

Lemon-Raspberry Soufflé

RATE QUALITY OF SLEEP:
(1 being the poorest and 5 being best)

1   (2)   3   4   5

RATE TODAY'S WHEAT TEMPTATION:
(5 being very strong cravings and 1 being no cravings at all)

1   2   3   (4)   5

RATE OVERALL MOOD:
(1 being the poorest and 5 being best)

1   2   (3)   4   5

ADDITIONAL COMMENTS/PROGRESS:

I was craving wheat less as the day progressed. Looking forward to a good

night's rest tonight!

WEEK 1—DAY 1

DATE:	WEIGHT:
BLOOD PRESSURE:	BLOOD SUGAR A.M./P.M.: /

BREAKFAST:

SNACK 1:

LUNCH:

SNACK 2:

DINNER:

SNACK 3:

RATE QUALITY OF SLEEP:
(1 being the poorest and 5 being best)

1	2	3	4	5

RATE TODAY'S WHEAT TEMPTATION:
(5 being very strong cravings and 1 being no cravings at all)

1	2	3	4	5

RATE OVERALL MOOD:
(1 being the poorest and 5 being best)

1	2	3	4	5

ADDITIONAL COMMENTS/PROGRESS:

_____

_____

_____

_____

_____

_____

_____

_____

_____

Reader Testimonial

"To any skeptics I would say, it's a simple enough experiment. Try it for a couple of weeks. See what happens."—Lucas (Wheat Belly Blog reader)

WEEK 1—DAY 2

DATE:	WEIGHT:
BLOOD PRESSURE:	BLOOD SUGAR A.M./P.M.: /

BREAKFAST:

SNACK 1:

LUNCH:

SNACK 2:

DINNER:

SNACK 3:

RATE QUALITY OF SLEEP:
(1 being the poorest and 5 being best)

1   2   3   4   5

RATE TODAY'S WHEAT TEMPTATION:
(5 being very strong cravings and 1 being no cravings at all)

1   2   3   4   5

RATE OVERALL MOOD:
(1 being the poorest and 5 being best)

1   2   3   4   5

ADDITIONAL COMMENTS/PROGRESS:

_____

_____

_____

_____

_____

_____

_____

_____

_____

_____

_____

_____

_____

WEEK 1—DAY 3

DATE:	WEIGHT:
BLOOD PRESSURE:	BLOOD SUGAR A.M./P.M.: /

BREAKFAST:

SNACK 1:

LUNCH:

SNACK 2:

DINNER:

SNACK 3:

RATE QUALITY OF SLEEP:
(1 being the poorest and 5 being best)

| 1 | 2 | 3 | 4 | 5 |

RATE TODAY'S WHEAT TEMPTATION:
(5 being very strong cravings and 1 being no cravings at all)

| 1 | 2 | 3 | 4 | 5 |

RATE OVERALL MOOD:
(1 being the poorest and 5 being best)

| 1 | 2 | 3 | 4 | 5 |

ADDITIONAL COMMENTS/PROGRESS:

_____

_____

_____

_____

_____

_____

_____

_____

_____

_____

_____

_____

_____

WEEK 1—DAY 4

DATE:	WEIGHT:
BLOOD PRESSURE:	BLOOD SUGAR A.M./P.M.: /

BREAKFAST:

SNACK 1:

LUNCH:

SNACK 2:

DINNER:

SNACK 3:

RATE QUALITY OF SLEEP:
(1 being the poorest and 5 being best)

1   2   3   4   5

RATE TODAY'S WHEAT TEMPTATION:
(5 being very strong cravings and 1 being no cravings at all)

1   2   3   4   5

RATE OVERALL MOOD:
(1 being the poorest and 5 being best)

1   2   3   4   5

ADDITIONAL COMMENTS/PROGRESS:

_____

_____

_____

_____

_____

_____

_____

_____

_____

_____

_____

_____

_____

WEEK 1—DAY 5

DATE:	WEIGHT:
BLOOD PRESSURE:	BLOOD SUGAR A.M./P.M.: /

BREAKFAST:

SNACK 1:

LUNCH:

SNACK 2:

DINNER:

SNACK 3:

RATE QUALITY OF SLEEP:
(1 being the poorest and 5 being best)

1	2	3	4	5

RATE TODAY'S WHEAT TEMPTATION:
(5 being very strong cravings and 1 being no cravings at all)

1	2	3	4	5

RATE OVERALL MOOD:
(1 being the poorest and 5 being best)

1	2	3	4	5

ADDITIONAL COMMENTS/PROGRESS:

WEEK 1—DAY 6

DATE:	WEIGHT:
BLOOD PRESSURE:	BLOOD SUGAR A.M./P.M.: /

BREAKFAST:

SNACK 1:

LUNCH:

SNACK 2:

DINNER:

SNACK 3:

RATE QUALITY OF SLEEP:
(1 being the poorest and 5 being best)

| 1 | 2 | 3 | 4 | 5 |

RATE TODAY'S WHEAT TEMPTATION:
(5 being very strong cravings and 1 being no cravings at all)

| 1 | 2 | 3 | 4 | 5 |

RATE OVERALL MOOD:
(1 being the poorest and 5 being best)

| 1 | 2 | 3 | 4 | 5 |

ADDITIONAL COMMENTS/PROGRESS:

_____

_____

_____

_____

_____

_____

_____

_____

_____

_____

_____

_____

_____

_____

WEEK 1—DAY 7

DATE:	WEIGHT:
BLOOD PRESSURE:	BLOOD SUGAR A.M./P.M.: /

BREAKFAST:

SNACK 1:

LUNCH:

SNACK 2:

DINNER:

SNACK 3:

RATE QUALITY OF SLEEP:
(1 being the poorest and 5 being best)

1	2	3	4	5

RATE TODAY'S WHEAT TEMPTATION:
(5 being very strong cravings and 1 being no cravings at all)

1	2	3	4	5

RATE OVERALL MOOD:
(1 being the poorest and 5 being best)

1	2	3	4	5

ADDITIONAL COMMENTS/PROGRESS:

_____

_____

_____

_____

_____

_____

_____

_____

_____

_____

_____

_____

_____

_____

Wheatopia

Just think of the enormity of the impact of wheat consumption on the human condition. Consumption of modern high-yield, semi-dwarf wheat leads to:

- **Weight gain**—especially visceral fat in the abdomen (i.e. inflammatory fat)
- **Diabetes, prediabetes**—via the appetite-stimulating effects of modern gliadin, the blood sugar–raising potential of amylopectin A, and the inflammatory effects of lectins
- **Hypertension**
- **Joint pain, arthritis**—mostly due to gliadin and wheat germ agglutinin
- **Gastrointestinal problems**—Acid reflux, irritable bowel syndrome, worsening symptoms of Crohn's disease and ulcerative colitis
- **Peripheral neuropathy, cerebellar ataxia, dementia**—due to gliadin
- **High cholesterol**—via increased triglycerides
- **Migraine headaches**—your guess is as good as mine why this occurs!
- **Depression**
- **Water retention, edema**—likely via the increased bowel and vascular permeability of lectins

And those are just the *common* phenomena. In fact, look at the list above and you will be hard pressed to find someone who is *not* afflicted with at least one, if not *all*, of the listed conditions. It means that much of what we do in healthcare such as treating diabetes, joint pain, and acid reflux is really just treating wheat consumption. We are treating the misguided advice to eat more "healthy whole grains."

Acid reflux alone afflicts some 60 million people and results in 100,000 hospitalizations every year. In my experience, it's a rare person who does not obtain total relief from acid reflux with wheat elimination. Eliminate wheat and watch hemoglobin A1c, the value that reflects your previous 60 days of blood sugar, plummet, converting many of the nation's 28 million diabetics and 70 million prediabetics to nondiabetics and non pre-diabetics.

While we fret about spiraling healthcare costs, the reorganization of healthcare delivery, and the deterioration of the health of Americans, there is an incredibly simple and accessible solution to a big chunk of the problem: Eliminate the wheat.

DEJA EWWW!

It's peculiar but instructive: re-exposure phenomena triggered by wheat exposure after being confidently wheat-free. The exposure can be intentional, as in "Just one won't hurt!" or it can be inadvertent, as in "That gravy looks okay." The most common re-exposure phenomena are:

- **Gastrointestinal distress,** bloating, and diarrhea that can last hours to a couple of days. (People with celiac disease can have problems for months, however.) This response resembles food poisoning.

- **Joint pain**—characteristically in the fingers and/or wrists

- **Upper airway phenomena** such as asthma and sinus congestion

- **Emotional effects** such as anxiety in females, irritability or rage in males

- **Appetite stimulation**—What I call the "I ate one cookie and gained 30 pounds" effect. Eating one cookie does not, of course, cause 30 pounds of weight gain. But just one exposure can set the appetite-stimulating machinery in motion and days or weeks of increased appetite for junk carbohydrates can result, thanks to the gliadin-derived opiates of wheat.

In addition, the symptoms that initially went away with your wheat-free adventure can return in all their glory. Like pushing a button, you can start or stop the process at will. It is a fitting reminder of just how inappropriate modern wheat is for humans.

WEEK 2—DAY 1

DATE:	WEIGHT:
BLOOD PRESSURE:	BLOOD SUGAR A.M./P.M.: /

BREAKFAST:

SNACK 1:

LUNCH:

SNACK 2:

DINNER:

SNACK 3:

RATE QUALITY OF SLEEP:
(1 being the poorest and 5 being best)

1	2	3	4	5

RATE TODAY'S WHEAT TEMPTATION:
(5 being very strong cravings and 1 being no cravings at all)

1	2	3	4	5

RATE OVERALL MOOD:
(1 being the poorest and 5 being best)

1	2	3	4	5

ADDITIONAL COMMENTS/PROGRESS:

_____

_____

_____

_____

_____

_____

Reader Tip

"I always tell people getting started to just pick a time frame of 2 to 3 weeks and just dive in and not commit beyond that. Believe it or not, for many people that is all it takes to reap many benefits—not just weight loss, but health benefits like improved skin, improved digestion, reduced or eliminated joint pain, and acid reflux elimination. A few weeks was all it took for me to decide I was never going back!"—Gary (Wheat Belly Blog reader)

WEEK 2—DAY 2

DATE:	WEIGHT:
BLOOD PRESSURE:	BLOOD SUGAR A.M./P.M.: /

BREAKFAST:

SNACK 1:

LUNCH:

SNACK 2:

DINNER:

SNACK 3:

RATE QUALITY OF SLEEP:
(1 being the poorest and 5 being best)

1	2	3	4	5

RATE TODAY'S WHEAT TEMPTATION:
(5 being very strong cravings and 1 being no cravings at all)

1	2	3	4	5

RATE OVERALL MOOD:
(1 being the poorest and 5 being best)

1	2	3	4	5

ADDITIONAL COMMENTS/PROGRESS:

_____

_____

_____

_____

_____

_____

_____

_____

_____

_____

_____

_____

_____

_____

WEEK 2—DAY 3

DATE:	WEIGHT:
BLOOD PRESSURE:	BLOOD SUGAR A.M./P.M.: /

BREAKFAST:

SNACK 1:

LUNCH:

SNACK 2:

DINNER:

SNACK 3:

RATE QUALITY OF SLEEP:
(1 being the poorest and 5 being best)

1	2	3	4	5

RATE TODAY'S WHEAT TEMPTATION:
(5 being very strong cravings and 1 being no cravings at all)

1	2	3	4	5

RATE OVERALL MOOD:
(1 being the poorest and 5 being best)

1	2	3	4	5

ADDITIONAL COMMENTS/PROGRESS:

_____

_____

_____

_____

_____

_____

_____

_____

_____

_____

_____

_____

_____

WEEK 2—DAY 4

DATE:	WEIGHT:
BLOOD PRESSURE:	BLOOD SUGAR A.M./P.M.: /

BREAKFAST:

SNACK 1:

LUNCH:

SNACK 2:

DINNER:

SNACK 3:

RATE QUALITY OF SLEEP:
(1 being the poorest and 5 being best)

1	2	3	4	5

RATE TODAY'S WHEAT TEMPTATION:
(5 being very strong cravings and 1 being no cravings at all)

1	2	3	4	5

RATE OVERALL MOOD:
(1 being the poorest and 5 being best)

1	2	3	4	5

ADDITIONAL COMMENTS/PROGRESS:

_____

_____

_____

_____

_____

_____

_____

_____

_____

_____

_____

_____

_____

_____

WEEK 2—DAY 5

DATE:	WEIGHT:
BLOOD PRESSURE:	BLOOD SUGAR A.M./P.M.: /

BREAKFAST:

SNACK 1:

LUNCH:

SNACK 2:

DINNER:

SNACK 3:

RATE QUALITY OF SLEEP:
(1 being the poorest and 5 being best)

| 1 | 2 | 3 | 4 | 5 |

RATE TODAY'S WHEAT TEMPTATION:
(5 being very strong cravings and 1 being no cravings at all)

| 1 | 2 | 3 | 4 | 5 |

RATE OVERALL MOOD:
(1 being the poorest and 5 being best)

| 1 | 2 | 3 | 4 | 5 |

ADDITIONAL COMMENTS/PROGRESS:

_____

_____

_____

_____

_____

_____

_____

_____

_____

_____

_____

_____

_____

WEEK 2—DAY 6

DATE:	WEIGHT:
BLOOD PRESSURE:	BLOOD SUGAR A.M./P.M.: /

BREAKFAST:

SNACK 1:

LUNCH:

SNACK 2:

DINNER:

SNACK 3:

RATE QUALITY OF SLEEP:
(1 being the poorest and 5 being best)

1   2   3   4   5

RATE TODAY'S WHEAT TEMPTATION:
(5 being very strong cravings and 1 being no cravings at all)

1   2   3   4   5

RATE OVERALL MOOD:
(1 being the poorest and 5 being best)

1   2   3   4   5

ADDITIONAL COMMENTS/PROGRESS:

_____

_____

_____

_____

_____

_____

_____

_____

_____

_____

_____

_____

_____

_____

_____

_____

WEEK 2—DAY 7

DATE:	WEIGHT:
BLOOD PRESSURE:	BLOOD SUGAR A.M./P.M.: /

BREAKFAST:

SNACK 1:

LUNCH:

SNACK 2:

DINNER:

SNACK 3:

RATE QUALITY OF SLEEP:
(1 being the poorest and 5 being best)

1   2   3   4   5

RATE TODAY'S WHEAT TEMPTATION:
(5 being very strong cravings and 1 being no cravings at all)

1   2   3   4   5

RATE OVERALL MOOD:
(1 being the poorest and 5 being best)

1   2   3   4   5

ADDITIONAL COMMENTS/PROGRESS:

_____

_____

_____

_____

_____

_____

_____

_____

_____

_____

_____

_____

_____

Corn Belly

 S ay you're starting from scratch and contemplating some changes to your diet. You suffer with heartburn, your joints hurt, your feet are swollen after standing on your feet for 8 hours. On your last visit to the doctor, your blood pressure was borderline high, your fasting blood sugar was in the pre-diabetic range, your cholesterol values were all screwed up, and your doctor threatened to put you on drugs for all of it unless you cut your calories and exercised more—even though you've been trying to push the plate away, consume smaller portions, and exercise vigorously at least 5 days a week.

So you decide to eliminate anything made of corn. This means you eliminate corn on the cob, any sauce or gravy thickened with cornstarch, tacos and tortillas or anything that might be made with cornmeal, and anything sweetened with high-fructose corn syrup. You continue to eat whole grain breads, pizza, and bagels. You try to limit your saturated fats and total fats. You eat plenty of fruits and vegetables.

What do you think happens?

Probably . . . nothing. Okay, so you lose 3 or 4 pounds, your fasting blood sugar drops from 112 mg/dl to 109 mg/dl, and your blood pressure drops from 140/90 to 137/84. After all, corn is an increasingly ubiquitous carbohydrate, and reducing your carbohydrate exposure can lead to such health benefits. Factor in the uncertainties introduced by genetically modified corn (glyphosate resistant and Bt toxin inoculated, in particular) and you have indeed achieved improvements in health.

But what about the other 70 pounds you've got to lose, the insatiable appetite, the still-high blood pressure and blood sugar, joint pains, peculiar rash on your arms and knees, leg edema, fatigue, depression, mental "fogginess," not to mention the behavioral problems of your 7-year-old, the acne of your 16-year-old, and the awkward and distressful cramps and diarrhea of your spouse?

You know where I'm going with this: It's *not* about corn. If the entire health mess most of us find ourselves in were about corn, well, then . . . eliminating corn would solve the entire collection of problems. It does not.

But eliminate the wheat, and an unexpected and broad range of health benefits develop. That's why the movement—not the book, but the *movement*—is labeled "Wheat Belly" and *not* corn belly, broccoli belly, beef belly, soda belly, high-fructose corn syrup belly, or any other belly.

It's called "Wheat Belly," and it's no mistake.

FAQ

Is wheat really that bad? I thought that whole grains were good for you?

First of all, it's not. It's the product of 40 years of genetics research aimed at increasing yield-per-acre. The result is a genetically unique plant that stands 2 feet tall, not the 4½-foot-tall "amber waves of grain" we all remember. The genetic distance modern wheat has drifted exceeds the difference between chimpanzees and humans. If you caught your son dating a chimpanzee, could you tell the difference? Of course you could! What a difference 1 percent can make. But that's more than modern wheat is removed from its ancestors.

WEEK 3—DAY 1

DATE:	WEIGHT:
BLOOD PRESSURE:	BLOOD SUGAR A.M./P.M.: /

BREAKFAST:

SNACK 1:

LUNCH:

SNACK 2:

DINNER:

SNACK 3:

RATE QUALITY OF SLEEP:
(1 being the poorest and 5 being best)

1	**2**	**3**	**4**	**5**

RATE TODAY'S WHEAT TEMPTATION:
(5 being very strong cravings and 1 being no cravings at all)

1	**2**	**3**	**4**	**5**

RATE OVERALL MOOD:
(1 being the poorest and 5 being best)

1	**2**	**3**	**4**	**5**

ADDITIONAL COMMENTS/PROGRESS:

_____

_____

_____

_____

_____

_____

_____

_____

Reader Testimonial

"After just 2 days, I could honestly say that I did not feel that heavy, bloated feeling like I was stuffed into my pants. It has been a little more than a week and for me the most wonderful feeling is a lighter feeling in my stomach: The heaviness is gone."—Ellie (Wheat Belly Blog reader)

WEEK 3—DAY 2

DATE:	WEIGHT:
BLOOD PRESSURE:	BLOOD SUGAR A.M./P.M.: /

BREAKFAST:

SNACK 1:

LUNCH:

SNACK 2:

DINNER:

SNACK 3:

RATE QUALITY OF SLEEP:
(1 being the poorest and 5 being best)

1	2	3	4	5

RATE TODAY'S WHEAT TEMPTATION:
(5 being very strong cravings and 1 being no cravings at all)

1	2	3	4	5

RATE OVERALL MOOD:
(1 being the poorest and 5 being best)

1	2	3	4	5

ADDITIONAL COMMENTS/PROGRESS:

_____

_____

_____

_____

_____

_____

_____

_____

_____

_____

_____

_____

_____

WEEK 3—DAY 3

DATE:	WEIGHT:
BLOOD PRESSURE:	BLOOD SUGAR A.M./P.M.: /

BREAKFAST:

SNACK 1:

LUNCH:

SNACK 2:

DINNER:

SNACK 3:

RATE QUALITY OF SLEEP:
(1 being the poorest and 5 being best)

1	2	3	4	5

RATE TODAY'S WHEAT TEMPTATION:
(5 being very strong cravings and 1 being no cravings at all)

1	2	3	4	5

RATE OVERALL MOOD:
(1 being the poorest and 5 being best)

1	2	3	4	5

ADDITIONAL COMMENTS/PROGRESS:

_____

_____

_____

_____

_____

_____

_____

_____

_____

_____

_____

_____

WEEK 3—DAY 4

DATE:	WEIGHT:
BLOOD PRESSURE:	BLOOD SUGAR A.M./P.M.: /

BREAKFAST:

SNACK 1:

LUNCH:

SNACK 2:

DINNER:

SNACK 3:

RATE QUALITY OF SLEEP:
(1 being the poorest and 5 being best)

| 1 | 2 | 3 | 4 | 5 |

RATE TODAY'S WHEAT TEMPTATION:
(5 being very strong cravings and 1 being no cravings at all)

| 1 | 2 | 3 | 4 | 5 |

RATE OVERALL MOOD:
(1 being the poorest and 5 being best)

| 1 | 2 | 3 | 4 | 5 |

ADDITIONAL COMMENTS/PROGRESS:

_____

_____

_____

_____

_____

_____

_____

_____

_____

_____

_____

_____

_____

WEEK 3—DAY 5

DATE:	WEIGHT:
BLOOD PRESSURE:	BLOOD SUGAR A.M./P.M.: /

BREAKFAST:

SNACK 1:

LUNCH:

SNACK 2:

DINNER:

SNACK 3:

RATE QUALITY OF SLEEP:
(1 being the poorest and 5 being best)

1	2	3	4	5

RATE TODAY'S WHEAT TEMPTATION:
(5 being very strong cravings and 1 being no cravings at all)

1	2	3	4	5

RATE OVERALL MOOD:
(1 being the poorest and 5 being best)

1	2	3	4	5

ADDITIONAL COMMENTS/PROGRESS:

_____

_____

_____

_____

_____

_____

_____

_____

_____

_____

_____

_____

_____

WEEK 3—DAY 6

DATE:	WEIGHT:
BLOOD PRESSURE:	BLOOD SUGAR A.M./P.M.: /

BREAKFAST:

SNACK 1:

LUNCH:

SNACK 2:

DINNER:

SNACK 3:

RATE QUALITY OF SLEEP:
(1 being the poorest and 5 being best)

| 1 | 2 | 3 | 4 | 5 |

RATE TODAY'S WHEAT TEMPTATION:
(5 being very strong cravings and 1 being no cravings at all)

| 1 | 2 | 3 | 4 | 5 |

RATE OVERALL MOOD:
(1 being the poorest and 5 being best)

| 1 | 2 | 3 | 4 | 5 |

ADDITIONAL COMMENTS/PROGRESS:

_____

_____

_____

_____

_____

_____

_____

_____

_____

_____

_____

_____

_____

_____

WEEK 3—DAY 7

DATE:	WEIGHT:
BLOOD PRESSURE:	BLOOD SUGAR A.M./P.M.: /

BREAKFAST:

SNACK 1:

LUNCH:

SNACK 2:

DINNER:

SNACK 3:

RATE QUALITY OF SLEEP:
(1 being the poorest and 5 being best)

| 1 | 2 | 3 | 4 | 5 |

RATE TODAY'S WHEAT TEMPTATION:
(5 being very strong cravings and 1 being no cravings at all)

| 1 | 2 | 3 | 4 | 5 |

RATE OVERALL MOOD:
(1 being the poorest and 5 being best)

| 1 | 2 | 3 | 4 | 5 |

ADDITIONAL COMMENTS/PROGRESS:

_____

_____

_____

_____

_____

_____

_____

_____

_____

_____

_____

_____

_____

Wheat-Eating Humans?

We modern humans, *Homo sapiens*, have walked the earth some 200,000 years. Our upright, bipedal, large-brained, and social hunter-gatherer predecessors, *Homo erectus*, walked the earth for nearly 10-fold longer, bridging the era when humans first began to eat animal flesh, whether via scavenging or hunting, and the relatively recent (500,000–700,000 years ago) harnessing of fire.

Before these two forms of *Homo*, we were preceded by *Homo habilis* (the "toolmaker"), believed to be the first to wield tools, and by the varieties of *Australopithecus*, harking back to a creature more ape-like, with longer, curved fingers and toes, less of an opposable thumb, brains that were much smaller, vertically longer pelvises, and longer arms and shorter legs than more recent versions of *Homo*. All these forms of human and pre-human reach back 10+ million years.

When was grain consumption, including wheat, added to the diet of humans? It wasn't during the time of *Australopithecus*, nor was it during the reign of *Homo habilis*. Although the long-successful *Homo erectus* learned how to scavenge/hunt animal flesh, they did not eat any wild-growing grains.

It wasn't until the last 5 percent of time since modern *Homo sapiens* appeared that they learned how to first harvest, then cultivate, wild wheat—known as einkorn. If we include the time of *Homo erectus*, then humans have consumed grains for only around 0.5 percent of the time they've walked the earth.

My point: Given the relatively slow process of evolution, we only need to look at the 2 million years of eating habits of *Homo erectus* and the first 190,000 or so years of *Homo sapiens* to recognize that consumption of grains like wheat is a very recent addition to the dietary habits of humans. For millions of years, humans evolved and survived without grains in any form.

Yes, harvesting of wild, then cultivated, grains provided the impetus for creating non-nomadic society and occupational specialization, a source of calories to supplement calories from animal products and plants. But is there any evolutionary or biologically plausible reason that we are now told that 60 percent or more of our calories should come from grains like wheat?

FAQ

Why do you make the claim that removing all wheat from the diet results in weight loss?

Because I've seen it happen—over and over and over again. It's lost from the deep visceral fat that resides within the abdomen, which are represented on the surface as "love handles" or a "muffin top"—what I call a "wheat belly." Typically, people who say goodbye to wheat lose a pound a day for the first 10 days. Weight loss then slows to yield 25 to 30 pounds over the subsequent 3 to 6 months (differing depending on body size, quality of diet at the start, male vs. female, etc.). When you remove wheat from the diet, you've removed a food that leads to fat deposition in the abdomen. Appetite diminishes, because the gliadin protein unique to wheat that is degraded to a morphine-like, appetite-stimulating compound is now gone. The average daily calorie intake drops 400 calories per day—with *less* hunger and *less* cravings, and food is more satisfying. This all occurs *without* imposing calorie limits, cutting fat grams, or limiting portion size. It all happens just by eliminating wheat.

WEEK 4—DAY 1

DATE:	WEIGHT:
BLOOD PRESSURE:	BLOOD SUGAR A.M./P.M.: /

BREAKFAST:

SNACK 1:

LUNCH:

SNACK 2:

DINNER:

SNACK 3:

RATE QUALITY OF SLEEP:
(1 being the poorest and 5 being best)

| 1 | 2 | 3 | 4 | 5 |

RATE TODAY'S WHEAT TEMPTATION:
(5 being very strong cravings and 1 being no cravings at all)

| 1 | 2 | 3 | 4 | 5 |

RATE OVERALL MOOD:
(1 being the poorest and 5 being best)

| 1 | 2 | 3 | 4 | 5 |

ADDITIONAL COMMENTS/PROGRESS:

_____

_____

_____

_____

_____

_____

_____

_____

Reader Tip

"At first I experienced some cravings, but I found that snacking on pecans left me satisfied."—Annemarie (Wheat Belly Blog reader)

WEEK 4—DAY 2

DATE:	WEIGHT:
BLOOD PRESSURE:	BLOOD SUGAR A.M./P.M.: /

BREAKFAST:

SNACK 1:

LUNCH:

SNACK 2:

DINNER:

SNACK 3:

RATE QUALITY OF SLEEP:
(1 being the poorest and 5 being best)

1   2   3   4   5

RATE TODAY'S WHEAT TEMPTATION:
(5 being very strong cravings and 1 being no cravings at all)

1   2   3   4   5

RATE OVERALL MOOD:
(1 being the poorest and 5 being best)

1   2   3   4   5

ADDITIONAL COMMENTS/PROGRESS:

WEEK 4—DAY 3

DATE:	WEIGHT:
BLOOD PRESSURE:	BLOOD SUGAR A.M./P.M.: /

BREAKFAST:

SNACK 1:

LUNCH:

SNACK 2:

DINNER:

SNACK 3:

RATE QUALITY OF SLEEP:
(1 being the poorest and 5 being best)

1	2	3	4	5

RATE TODAY'S WHEAT TEMPTATION:
(5 being very strong cravings and 1 being no cravings at all)

1	2	3	4	5

RATE OVERALL MOOD:
(1 being the poorest and 5 being best)

1	2	3	4	5

ADDITIONAL COMMENTS/PROGRESS:

_____

_____

_____

_____

_____

_____

_____

_____

_____

_____

_____

_____

_____

WEEK 4—DAY 4

DATE:	WEIGHT:
BLOOD PRESSURE:	BLOOD SUGAR A.M./P.M.: /

BREAKFAST:

SNACK 1:

LUNCH:

SNACK 2:

DINNER:

SNACK 3:

RATE QUALITY OF SLEEP:
(1 being the poorest and 5 being best)

1	2	3	4	5

RATE TODAY'S WHEAT TEMPTATION:
(5 being very strong cravings and 1 being no cravings at all)

1	2	3	4	5

RATE OVERALL MOOD:
(1 being the poorest and 5 being best)

1	2	3	4	5

ADDITIONAL COMMENTS/PROGRESS:

_____

_____

_____

_____

_____

_____

_____

_____

_____

_____

_____

_____

_____

_____

_____

WEEK 4—DAY 5

DATE:	WEIGHT:
BLOOD PRESSURE:	BLOOD SUGAR A.M./P.M.: /

BREAKFAST:

SNACK 1:

LUNCH:

SNACK 2:

DINNER:

SNACK 3:

RATE QUALITY OF SLEEP:
(1 being the poorest and 5 being best)

| 1 | 2 | 3 | 4 | 5 |

RATE TODAY'S WHEAT TEMPTATION:
(5 being very strong cravings and 1 being no cravings at all)

| 1 | 2 | 3 | 4 | 5 |

RATE OVERALL MOOD:
(1 being the poorest and 5 being best)

| 1 | 2 | 3 | 4 | 5 |

ADDITIONAL COMMENTS/PROGRESS:

WEEK 4—DAY 6

DATE:	WEIGHT:
BLOOD PRESSURE:	BLOOD SUGAR A.M./P.M.: /

BREAKFAST:

SNACK 1:

LUNCH:

SNACK 2:

DINNER:

SNACK 3:

RATE QUALITY OF SLEEP:
(1 being the poorest and 5 being best)

| 1 | 2 | 3 | 4 | 5 |

RATE TODAY'S WHEAT TEMPTATION:
(5 being very strong cravings and 1 being no cravings at all)

| 1 | 2 | 3 | 4 | 5 |

RATE OVERALL MOOD:
(1 being the poorest and 5 being best)

| 1 | 2 | 3 | 4 | 5 |

ADDITIONAL COMMENTS/PROGRESS:

_____

_____

_____

_____

_____

_____

_____

_____

_____

_____

_____

_____

_____

_____

WEEK 4—DAY 7

DATE:	WEIGHT:
BLOOD PRESSURE:	BLOOD SUGAR A.M./P.M.: /

BREAKFAST:

SNACK 1:

LUNCH:

SNACK 2:

DINNER:

SNACK 3:

RATE QUALITY OF SLEEP:
(1 being the poorest and 5 being best)

1	2	3	4	5

RATE TODAY'S WHEAT TEMPTATION:
(5 being very strong cravings and 1 being no cravings at all)

1	2	3	4	5

RATE OVERALL MOOD:
(1 being the poorest and 5 being best)

1	2	3	4	5

ADDITIONAL COMMENTS/PROGRESS:

_____

_____

_____

_____

_____

_____

_____

_____

_____

_____

_____

_____

_____

Hunger Pangs

Eliminate modern high-yield, semi-dwarf *Triticum aestivum* . . . and what is the effect on appetite?

A reduction in appetite is among the most common and profound experiences resulting from wheat elimination. I know that I have felt it: Wake up in the morning and have little interest in breakfast for several hours. Lunch? Maybe I'll have a few bites of something. Dinner . . . well, I'd like to exercise first.

The wheatless report that:

- Appetite diminishes to the point where you can't remember whether you've eaten or not. It is not uncommon to miss a meal—and feel perfectly content. Calorie intake drops by *400 calories per day*, on average calories you otherwise would not have needed but all went to your stomach.

- Hunger *feels* different: It's not the gnawing, rumbling hunger that plagues you every 2 hours. In its place, you will find that hunger feels like a soft reminder that maybe it's time to have something to eat because you haven't had anything in—what?—4 to 6 hours. And it's a subtle reminder, not a desperate hunt that makes you knock people aside at the food bar, steal coworkers' lunches stored in the refrigerator, or salivate at the mere thought of food.

- The simplest foods satisfy—it no longer requires an all-you-can-eat buffet to satisfy, but a few small pieces of healthy food. (Yes, but what happens to revenues at Kraft, Nabisco, and Kellogg's, not to mention the revenues at agribusiness giants ADM and Monsanto? Slash consumption by, say, 30%, you likewise slash revenues by 30%. What would shareholders say?)

- Even prolonged periods of not eating, i.e., fasting, are endured with ease.

Hunger and the relentless search for something to eat disappear for most people. By eliminating the appetite-stimulating properties of wheat, we return to a natural state of eating for sustenance, to satisfy physiologic need. We are no longer victims of this incredibly powerful appetite stimulant called *gliadin* from wheat.

This is why many diets fail: They fail to remove this powerful appetite stimulant. You might eat only lean meats, limit your calories, and exercise 90 minutes per day, but as long as the gliadin protein is pushing your appetite button, you will want to eat more or you will have to mount monumental willpower to resist it.

So the key is to remove the gliadin protein from your life by eliminate all things wheat.

FAQ

When you examine food labels in the grocery store, you see that wheat is in nearly everything. Is it really practical to remove all wheat from the diet?

Yes, it is. It means a return to *real* food from the produce aisle, fish and meat department, nuts, eggs, olives, and oils.

This question raises another crucial one: Just *why* is wheat such a ubiquitous ingredient in so many foods, from ice cream to french fries? That's easy: Because it tastes good and it stimulates appetite. You want more wheat, you want more of everything else to the tune of 400 or more calories per day. More calories, more food, and, therefore, more revenue for Big Food. Wheat is not in cucumbers, green peppers, salmon, or walnuts. But it's in over 90 percent of the foods on supermarket shelves, all there to stimulate your appetite center to consume more . . . and more and more.

Living wheat-free means being equipped with recipes that allow you to re-create familiar recipes that you might miss, like cheesecake, cookies, and biscotti—without wheat, with little to no sugar or carbohydrate exposure, yet healthy. That's what I've done in *Wheat Belly*.

WEEK 5—DAY 1

DATE:	WEIGHT:
BLOOD PRESSURE:	BLOOD SUGAR A.M./P.M.: /

BREAKFAST:

SNACK 1:

LUNCH:

SNACK 2:

DINNER:

SNACK 3:

RATE QUALITY OF SLEEP:
(1 being the poorest and 5 being best)

| 1 | 2 | 3 | 4 | 5 |

RATE TODAY'S WHEAT TEMPTATION:
(5 being very strong cravings and 1 being no cravings at all)

| 1 | 2 | 3 | 4 | 5 |

RATE OVERALL MOOD:
(1 being the poorest and 5 being best)

| 1 | 2 | 3 | 4 | 5 |

ADDITIONAL COMMENTS/PROGRESS:

_____

_____

_____

_____

_____

_____

_____

Reader Testimonial

"In 6 weeks I have lost 10 pounds, lost 4 inches in my waist, my cholesterol has dropped from 206 (stable on statins) to 125, my LDL decreased and my HDL increased. I stopped my twice a day GERD medicine. I was able to drop one blood pressure medication (HCTZ) and decrease the dose in the second (Benicar). And the very best thing of all is that I no longer have food cravings, I no longer binge! What a victory!"—Linda (Wheat Belly Blog reader)

WEEK 5—DAY 2

DATE:	WEIGHT:
BLOOD PRESSURE:	BLOOD SUGAR A.M./P.M.: /

BREAKFAST:

SNACK 1:

LUNCH:

SNACK 2:

DINNER:

SNACK 3:

RATE QUALITY OF SLEEP:
(1 being the poorest and 5 being best)

1	2	3	4	5

RATE TODAY'S WHEAT TEMPTATION:
(5 being very strong cravings and 1 being no cravings at all)

1	2	3	4	5

RATE OVERALL MOOD:
(1 being the poorest and 5 being best)

1	2	3	4	5

ADDITIONAL COMMENTS/PROGRESS:

_____

_____

_____

_____

_____

_____

_____

_____

_____

_____

_____

_____

WEEK 5—DAY 3

DATE:	WEIGHT:
BLOOD PRESSURE:	BLOOD SUGAR A.M./P.M.: /

BREAKFAST:

SNACK 1:

LUNCH:

SNACK 2:

DINNER:

SNACK 3:

RATE QUALITY OF SLEEP:
(1 being the poorest and 5 being best)

1	2	3	4	5

RATE TODAY'S WHEAT TEMPTATION:
(5 being very strong cravings and 1 being no cravings at all)

1	2	3	4	5

RATE OVERALL MOOD:
(1 being the poorest and 5 being best)

1	2	3	4	5

ADDITIONAL COMMENTS/PROGRESS:

_____

_____

_____

_____

_____

_____

_____

_____

_____

_____

_____

_____

WEEK 5—DAY 4

DATE:	WEIGHT:
BLOOD PRESSURE:	BLOOD SUGAR A.M./P.M.: /

BREAKFAST:

SNACK 1:

LUNCH:

SNACK 2:

DINNER:

SNACK 3:

RATE QUALITY OF SLEEP:
(1 being the poorest and 5 being best)

1	2	3	4	5

RATE TODAY'S WHEAT TEMPTATION:
(5 being very strong cravings and 1 being no cravings at all)

1	2	3	4	5

RATE OVERALL MOOD:
(1 being the poorest and 5 being best)

1	2	3	4	5

ADDITIONAL COMMENTS/PROGRESS:

_____

_____

_____

_____

_____

_____

_____

_____

_____

_____

_____

_____

WEEK 5—DAY 5

DATE:	WEIGHT:
BLOOD PRESSURE:	BLOOD SUGAR A.M./P.M.: /

BREAKFAST:

SNACK 1:

LUNCH:

SNACK 2:

DINNER:

SNACK 3:

RATE QUALITY OF SLEEP:
(1 being the poorest and 5 being best)

1	2	3	4	5

RATE TODAY'S WHEAT TEMPTATION:
(5 being very strong cravings and 1 being no cravings at all)

1	2	3	4	5

RATE OVERALL MOOD:
(1 being the poorest and 5 being best)

1	2	3	4	5

ADDITIONAL COMMENTS/PROGRESS:

_____

_____

_____

_____

_____

_____

_____

_____

_____

_____

_____

_____

WEEK 5—DAY 6

DATE:	WEIGHT:
BLOOD PRESSURE:	BLOOD SUGAR A.M./P.M.: /

BREAKFAST:

SNACK 1:

LUNCH:

SNACK 2:

DINNER:

SNACK 3:

RATE QUALITY OF SLEEP:
(1 being the poorest and 5 being best)

1	2	3	4	5

RATE TODAY'S WHEAT TEMPTATION:
(5 being very strong cravings and 1 being no cravings at all)

1	2	3	4	5

RATE OVERALL MOOD:
(1 being the poorest and 5 being best)

1	2	3	4	5

ADDITIONAL COMMENTS/PROGRESS:

_____

_____

_____

_____

_____

_____

_____

_____

_____

_____

_____

_____

_____

_____

WEEK 5—DAY 7

DATE:	WEIGHT:
BLOOD PRESSURE:	BLOOD SUGAR A.M./P.M.: /

BREAKFAST:

SNACK 1:

LUNCH:

SNACK 2:

DINNER:

SNACK 3:

RATE QUALITY OF SLEEP:
(1 being the poorest and 5 being best)

1	2	3	4	5

RATE TODAY'S WHEAT TEMPTATION:
(5 being very strong cravings and 1 being no cravings at all)

1	2	3	4	5

RATE OVERALL MOOD:
(1 being the poorest and 5 being best)

1	2	3	4	5

ADDITIONAL COMMENTS/PROGRESS:

_____

_____

_____

_____

_____

_____

_____

_____

_____

_____

_____

_____

Unapproved Drugs

Imagine a world in which the pharmaceutical industry were permitted to develop drugs, then bring them directly to market, no regulatory process required. They develop a drug to treat a specific condition, like toe fungus or depression, then introduce it to market for pharmacies to sell and physicians to promote, no FDA application required. The developer might have performed the usual phase 1, 2, and 3 clinical trials, they might not have. They can just bring it to market, no questions asked about safety, efficacy, or suitability for human consumption.

Imagine the mess that would result. It would be pure profiteering and marketing.

While the FDA process is far from perfect, it does introduce a level of scrutiny, a requirement to test for safety and, to some degree, efficacy. Anyone who has contributed to these sorts of trials or seen the incredible reams of paperwork filed for an FDA New Drug Application knows how demanding these requirements can be.

There is no such requirement for food crops widely consumed by humans.

In effect, 50 years of plant hybridization, crossbreeding, backcrossing, chemical and radiation mutagenesis (induction of mutations), and now gene splicing ("genetic modification") have allowed the appearance of new compounds in food crops, most of which have not been studied but are widely consumed by humans. Agricultural genetics has, in effect, permitted the appearance of multiple new "drugs" on the market without any regulatory scrutiny or safety testing in animals or humans. The result: Commercial foods that have poorly-understood effects on humans.

So, yes, modern food mistakes are about such issues as overconsumption of sucrose, overexposure to fructose, food colorings and preservatives, and relative macronutrient intake (e.g., excessive carbohydrate intake). But it's also about the substantial changes introduced into food crops like wheat, corn, and soy that have not been examined—*because the questions were never asked.*

FAQ

What exactly is in wheat that makes it so bad?

Gluten is only one of the reasons to fear wheat, since it triggers a host of immune diseases like celiac, rheumatoid arthritis, and gluten encephalopathy (dementia from wheat).

The protein unique to wheat, gliadin, a component of gluten proteins, is odd in that it is degraded in the human gastrointestinal tract to polypeptides (small proteins) that have the ability to cross into the brain and bind to morphine receptors. These polypeptides have been labeled *gluteomorphins* or *exorphins* (exogenous morphine-like compounds) by National Institutes of Health researchers. Wheat exorphins cause a subtle euphoria in some people. This may be part of the reason wheat products increase appetite and cause addiction-like behaviors in susceptible people. It also explains why a drug company has made application to the FDA for the drug naltrexone, an oral opiate-blocking drug ordinarily used to keep heroin addicts drug free, for weight loss. Block the brain morphine receptor, and weight loss (about 22 pounds over 6 months) results. But there's only one food that yields substantial morphine-like compounds: wheat.

The complex carbohydrate unique to wheat, amylopectin A, is another problem source. The branching structure of wheat's amylopectin A is more digestible than the amylopectins B and C from rice, beans, and other starches (i.e., in their natural states, not the gluten-free dried pulverized starches). This explains why two slices of whole wheat bread increase blood sugar higher than table sugar, higher than a bowl of brown rice, higher than many candy bars. Ingesting high blood sugars repeatedly is not good for health. It leads to accumulated visceral fat—a "wheat belly," diabetes and prediabetes (defined, of course, as having higher blood sugars), not to mention cataracts, arthritis, and heart disease.

As if that wasn't enough, even other components of wheat are harmful, such as the lectins in wheat. The lectin unique to wheat is wheat germ agglutinin, a *direct intestinal toxin* that exerts destructive effects on the lining and can even mimic the damage of celiac disease.

WEEK 6—DAY 1

DATE:	WEIGHT:
BLOOD PRESSURE:	BLOOD SUGAR A.M./P.M.: /

BREAKFAST:

SNACK 1:

LUNCH:

SNACK 2:

DINNER:

SNACK 3:

RATE QUALITY OF SLEEP:
(1 being the poorest and 5 being best)

| 1 | 2 | 3 | 4 | 5 |

RATE TODAY'S WHEAT TEMPTATION:
(5 being very strong cravings and 1 being no cravings at all)

| 1 | 2 | 3 | 4 | 5 |

RATE OVERALL MOOD:
(1 being the poorest and 5 being best)

| 1 | 2 | 3 | 4 | 5 |

ADDITIONAL COMMENTS/PROGRESS:

_____

_____

_____

_____

_____

_____

_____

_____

Reader Testimonial

"My life is so different now. I have more energy than ever, and am so hopeful and excited knowing that my next 48 years will be filled with active adventure and fun, instead of doctor's visits, statin drugs, diabetes, and stiff and achy joints."—Gary (Wheat Belly Blog reader)

WEEK 6—DAY 2

DATE:	WEIGHT:
BLOOD PRESSURE:	BLOOD SUGAR A.M./P.M.: /

BREAKFAST:

SNACK 1:

LUNCH:

SNACK 2:

DINNER:

SNACK 3:

RATE QUALITY OF SLEEP:
(1 being the poorest and 5 being best)

1	2	3	4	5

RATE TODAY'S WHEAT TEMPTATION:
(5 being very strong cravings and 1 being no cravings at all)

1	2	3	4	5

RATE OVERALL MOOD:
(1 being the poorest and 5 being best)

1	2	3	4	5

ADDITIONAL COMMENTS/PROGRESS:

_____

_____

_____

_____

_____

_____

_____

_____

_____

_____

_____

_____

WEEK 6—DAY 3

DATE:	WEIGHT:
BLOOD PRESSURE:	BLOOD SUGAR A.M./P.M.: /

BREAKFAST:

SNACK 1:

LUNCH:

SNACK 2:

DINNER:

SNACK 3:

RATE QUALITY OF SLEEP:
(1 being the poorest and 5 being best)

1   2   3   4   5

RATE TODAY'S WHEAT TEMPTATION:
(5 being very strong cravings and 1 being no cravings at all)

1   2   3   4   5

RATE OVERALL MOOD:
(1 being the poorest and 5 being best)

1   2   3   4   5

ADDITIONAL COMMENTS/PROGRESS:

_____

_____

_____

_____

_____

_____

_____

_____

_____

_____

_____

_____

_____

WEEK 6—DAY 4

DATE:	WEIGHT:
BLOOD PRESSURE:	BLOOD SUGAR A.M./P.M.: /

BREAKFAST:

SNACK 1:

LUNCH:

SNACK 2:

DINNER:

SNACK 3:

RATE QUALITY OF SLEEP:
(1 being the poorest and 5 being best)

1	2	3	4	5

RATE TODAY'S WHEAT TEMPTATION:
(5 being very strong cravings and 1 being no cravings at all)

1	2	3	4	5

RATE OVERALL MOOD:
(1 being the poorest and 5 being best)

1	2	3	4	5

ADDITIONAL COMMENTS/PROGRESS:

WEEK 6—DAY 5

DATE:	WEIGHT:
BLOOD PRESSURE:	BLOOD SUGAR A.M./P.M.: /

BREAKFAST:

SNACK 1:

LUNCH:

SNACK 2:

DINNER:

SNACK 3:

RATE QUALITY OF SLEEP:
(1 being the poorest and 5 being best)

1	2	3	4	5

RATE TODAY'S WHEAT TEMPTATION:
(5 being very strong cravings and 1 being no cravings at all)

1	2	3	4	5

RATE OVERALL MOOD:
(1 being the poorest and 5 being best)

1	2	3	4	5

ADDITIONAL COMMENTS/PROGRESS:

_____

_____

_____

_____

_____

_____

_____

_____

_____

_____

_____

_____

_____

_____

WEEK 6—DAY 6

DATE:	WEIGHT:
BLOOD PRESSURE:	BLOOD SUGAR A.M./P.M.: /

BREAKFAST:

SNACK 1:

LUNCH:

SNACK 2:

DINNER:

SNACK 3:

RATE QUALITY OF SLEEP:
(1 being the poorest and 5 being best)

1	2	3	4	5

RATE TODAY'S WHEAT TEMPTATION:
(5 being very strong cravings and 1 being no cravings at all)

1	2	3	4	5

RATE OVERALL MOOD:
(1 being the poorest and 5 being best)

1	2	3	4	5

ADDITIONAL COMMENTS/PROGRESS:

_____

_____

_____

_____

_____

_____

_____

_____

_____

_____

_____

_____

_____

WEEK 6—DAY 7

DATE:	WEIGHT:
BLOOD PRESSURE:	BLOOD SUGAR A.M./P.M.: /

BREAKFAST:

SNACK 1:

LUNCH:

SNACK 2:

DINNER:

SNACK 3:

RATE QUALITY OF SLEEP:
(1 being the poorest and 5 being best)

1	2	3	4	5

RATE TODAY'S WHEAT TEMPTATION:
(5 being very strong cravings and 1 being no cravings at all)

1	2	3	4	5

RATE OVERALL MOOD:
(1 being the poorest and 5 being best)

1	2	3	4	5

ADDITIONAL COMMENTS/PROGRESS:

Almonds are the New Wheat

Once you eliminate the genetically-altered Frankengrain called modern wheat, your diet should center around vegetables, nuts, healthy oils like olive and coconut, fish, meats, cheese, olives, avocados, and other real whole foods. This is the diet that I have advocated in my heart disease prevention practice, as well as my online program for prevention and reversal of heart disease.

But what if you'd like a piece of cheesecake or a nice slice of dessert bread? You don't want to gain two pounds, spend 48 hours in the bathroom suffering with diarrhea and cramps, deal with 3 weeks of joint pains and leg swelling, wade through mental "fog," anxiety, and rage just because you had that momentary indulgence—as you would with wheat?

That's why I focus on recipes that allow you to have something familiar, such as chocolate coconut bread or biscotti, by using ingredients that will *not* generate the metabolic contortions triggered by wheat.

On perusing the recipes in *Wheat Belly Cookbook*, you will notice that there are recurring ingredient themes. Many of the same ingredients pop up time and again. Among the most frequent, versatile, user-friendly, and tasty: Almonds.

Various types of almonds include ground whole almonds, ground blanched almonds for a finer texture, ground roasted almonds, and almond butter (though, for maximum health benefits, I prefer ground whole almonds). Ground almonds allow you to re-create muffins, breads, scones, pizza crust, pie crust, biscotti, and cookies with health benefits that *exceed* that of whole wheat—but with *none* of the downside: no weight gain, no high blood sugar, no triggering of small LDL particles (the number one cause of heart disease in the U.S.), no accumulation of visceral fat, and no appetite stimulation.

In short, you can have your chocolate-almond biscotti or mocha cupcake and enjoy it, no health price to pay. So I call almonds the new wheat, except better.

FAQ

If I go wheat free, is there any harm in having an occasional bagel or cupcake?

It depends on your individual susceptibility to the effects of wheat.

If you have celiac disease or any of the long list of inflammatory or autoimmune diseases associated with wheat (rheumatoid arthritis, cerebellar ataxia, peripheral neuropathy, Hashimoto's thyroiditis, dermatitis herpetiformis, etc.), then wheat and gluten avoidance should be complete and meticulous.

If you have an addictive relationship with wheat, such that one pretzel makes you want to eat the whole bag, then complete avoidance is also advisable. Because the 30 percent of people with this problem cannot stop consuming wheat once they start, it is best to avoid wheat-containing foods altogether.

Yet another odd observation: Many, though not all, people who have removed wheat from their diet for at least several months have what I call "wheat reexposure reactions." They may experience abdominal cramps, gas, and diarrhea (just like food poisoning); asthma attacks in the susceptible; joint swelling and pain; and emotional effects such as anxiety in women and rage in men. I've witnessed many people go wheat free, feel great, lose 30 pounds, then have an emotional blowup at a birthday party after indulging in just a small piece of birthday cake, and then spending the next 24 hours on the toilet with diarrhea.

There are indeed a percentage (20 to 30 percent) of people who can get away with occasional indulgences. Sometimes it's a matter of running a little test yourself to gauge your reaction. Anyone with a history of autoimmune or inflammatory diseases, or having had celiac markers like an anti-gliadin antibody test positive, however, should not even try this.

WEEK 7—DAY 1

DATE:	WEIGHT:
BLOOD PRESSURE:	BLOOD SUGAR A.M./P.M.: /

BREAKFAST:

SNACK 1:

LUNCH:

SNACK 2:

DINNER:

SNACK 3:

RATE QUALITY OF SLEEP:
(1 being the poorest and 5 being best)

1	2	3	4	5

RATE TODAY'S WHEAT TEMPTATION:
(5 being very strong cravings and 1 being no cravings at all)

1	2	3	4	5

RATE OVERALL MOOD:
(1 being the poorest and 5 being best)

1	2	3	4	5

ADDITIONAL COMMENTS/PROGRESS:

_____

_____

_____

_____

_____

_____

_____

Wheat Belly Tip

"After four days on this wheat-free program, I was feeling very light around my stomach and I thought, 'Well, for today I can cheat and just have one biscotti with my coffee.' HOW WRONG I WAS. Just that one biscotti and I felt like I had cement in my stomach. Never again. I never realized what wheat can do to you. Back on track I went."—Ellie (Wheat Belly Blog reader)

WEEK 7—DAY 2

DATE:	WEIGHT:
BLOOD PRESSURE:	BLOOD SUGAR A.M./P.M.: /

BREAKFAST:

SNACK 1:

LUNCH:

SNACK 2:

DINNER:

SNACK 3:

RATE QUALITY OF SLEEP:
(1 being the poorest and 5 being best)

| 1 | 2 | 3 | 4 | 5 |

RATE TODAY'S WHEAT TEMPTATION:
(5 being very strong cravings and 1 being no cravings at all)

| 1 | 2 | 3 | 4 | 5 |

RATE OVERALL MOOD:
(1 being the poorest and 5 being best)

| 1 | 2 | 3 | 4 | 5 |

ADDITIONAL COMMENTS/PROGRESS:

_____

_____

_____

_____

_____

_____

_____

_____

_____

_____

_____

_____

_____

_____

WEEK 7—DAY 3

DATE:	WEIGHT:
BLOOD PRESSURE:	BLOOD SUGAR A.M./P.M.: /

BREAKFAST:

SNACK 1:

LUNCH:

SNACK 2:

DINNER:

SNACK 3:

RATE QUALITY OF SLEEP:
(1 being the poorest and 5 being best)

1	2	3	4	5

RATE TODAY'S WHEAT TEMPTATION:
(5 being very strong cravings and 1 being no cravings at all)

1	2	3	4	5

RATE OVERALL MOOD:
(1 being the poorest and 5 being best)

1	2	3	4	5

ADDITIONAL COMMENTS/PROGRESS:

_____

_____

_____

_____

_____

_____

_____

_____

_____

_____

_____

_____

_____

WEEK 7—DAY 4

DATE:	WEIGHT:
BLOOD PRESSURE:	BLOOD SUGAR A.M./P.M.: /

BREAKFAST:

SNACK 1:

LUNCH:

SNACK 2:

DINNER:

SNACK 3:

RATE QUALITY OF SLEEP:
(1 being the poorest and 5 being best)

| 1 | 2 | 3 | 4 | 5 |

RATE TODAY'S WHEAT TEMPTATION:
(5 being very strong cravings and 1 being no cravings at all)

| 1 | 2 | 3 | 4 | 5 |

RATE OVERALL MOOD:
(1 being the poorest and 5 being best)

| 1 | 2 | 3 | 4 | 5 |

ADDITIONAL COMMENTS/PROGRESS:

_____

_____

_____

_____

_____

_____

_____

_____

_____

_____

_____

_____

WEEK 7—DAY 5

DATE:	WEIGHT:
BLOOD PRESSURE:	BLOOD SUGAR A.M./P.M.: /

BREAKFAST:

SNACK 1:

LUNCH:

SNACK 2:

DINNER:

SNACK 3:

RATE QUALITY OF SLEEP:
(1 being the poorest and 5 being best)

1	2	3	4	5

RATE TODAY'S WHEAT TEMPTATION:
(5 being very strong cravings and 1 being no cravings at all)

1	2	3	4	5

RATE OVERALL MOOD:
(1 being the poorest and 5 being best)

1	2	3	4	5

ADDITIONAL COMMENTS/PROGRESS:

_____

_____

_____

_____

_____

_____

_____

_____

_____

_____

_____

_____

_____

WEEK 7—DAY 6

DATE:	WEIGHT:
BLOOD PRESSURE:	BLOOD SUGAR A.M./P.M.: /

BREAKFAST:

SNACK 1:

LUNCH:

SNACK 2:

DINNER:

SNACK 3:

RATE QUALITY OF SLEEP:
(1 being the poorest and 5 being best)

| 1 | 2 | 3 | 4 | 5 |

RATE TODAY'S WHEAT TEMPTATION:
(5 being very strong cravings and 1 being no cravings at all)

| 1 | 2 | 3 | 4 | 5 |

RATE OVERALL MOOD:
(1 being the poorest and 5 being best)

| 1 | 2 | 3 | 4 | 5 |

ADDITIONAL COMMENTS/PROGRESS:

_____

_____

_____

_____

_____

_____

_____

_____

_____

_____

_____

_____

_____

WEEK 7—DAY 7

DATE:	WEIGHT:
BLOOD PRESSURE:	BLOOD SUGAR A.M./P.M.: /

BREAKFAST:

SNACK 1:

LUNCH:

SNACK 2:

DINNER:

SNACK 3:

RATE QUALITY OF SLEEP:
(1 being the poorest and 5 being best)

| 1 | 2 | 3 | 4 | 5 |

RATE TODAY'S WHEAT TEMPTATION:
(5 being very strong cravings and 1 being no cravings at all)

| 1 | 2 | 3 | 4 | 5 |

RATE OVERALL MOOD:
(1 being the poorest and 5 being best)

| 1 | 2 | 3 | 4 | 5 |

ADDITIONAL COMMENTS/PROGRESS:

_____

_____

_____

_____

_____

_____

_____

_____

_____

_____

_____

_____

_____

How Sweet It Is!

D oes wheat cause diabetes? Is the national message to eat more "healthy whole grains" to blame for the nationwide epidemic of diabetes? Can that bowl of bran cereal, English muffin, or plate of whole wheat pasta mean a life of drugs, insulin injections, and eight years shaved off your lifespan?

Yes, yes, and yes. Mind you, I am a vigorous advocate of the elimination of all wheat from the human diet. Even without hearing the rationale for this opinion, many people are experiencing substantial weight loss and health turnarounds by eliminating wheat. But can we blame *diabetes* on wheat?

Yes, absolutely. There are several reasons why wheat, more than many other foods, causes diabetes:

- Any food that increases blood sugar to high levels also increases insulin to high levels. Repetitive high insulin leads to *insulin resistance*, which leads to visceral fat deposition, more insulin resistance, inflammation, etc., eventuating in diabetes.

- High blood sugar, such as that resulting from eating whole wheat bread, is toxic to pancreatic beta cells, the cells that produce insulin: *glucotoxicity*.

- Triglyceride-containing lipoproteins, such as chylomicrons and its remnants, are toxic to pancreatic beta cells: *lipotoxicity*.

- The gliadin protein of wheat stimulates appetite, causing the unwitting wheat consumer to eat, on average, 400 more calories per day, mostly from carbohydrates. Four hundred calories per day, 365 days per year . . . that's a lot of extra calories and a lot of potential weight gain.

- The lectins of wheat (wheat germ agglutinin) generate inflammation in multiple sites, such as joints, the intestinal tract, and endocrine glands. And higher levels of inflammation (and its various mediators) worsen insulin resistance.

Some aspects of wheat (especially gliadin and lectins) became much worse with the introduction of modern high-yield, semi-dwarf strains of wheat, compounded with the advice to cut your fat and eat more "healthy whole grains." This deadly combination coincided precisely with the beginning of the explosion in diabetes in the U.S.

Sugars and processed foods made of such things as cornstarch and high-fructose corn syrup also make a major contribution. But they lack the direct inflammatory effects of lectins and the appetite-stimulating effects of gliadin. They are bad, but do not compare to the effects of this thing called "wheat."

High-yield, semi-dwarf wheat was introduced into the U.S. in the mid-1970s. By 1985, virtually all bagels, pizza, and bread originated with this darling of agricultural geneticists. The new gliadin of wheat (altered by several amino acids), a more effective appetite stimulant than its predecessor, "old" gliadin, caused calorie consumption to increase by 400 to 500 calories per day. Americans gained weight. A several-year lag followed before the uptick in diabetes began, as it requires 30, 40, 50, or more pounds for most people to exhibit all the hallmarks of diabetes.

So we now have the world's worst epidemic of diabetes ever witnessed since humans have walked on earth. Some "experts" argue that it's genetics or the overconsumption of soda. Others argue that it's physical inactivity, lives spent behind desks, looking at computer screens.

I personally became diabetic 20 years ago at a time when I was jogging 3 to 5 miles per day, cutting my fat, avoiding junk foods and soft drinks, and eating plenty of "healthy whole grains." But I became diabetic. I believe this is the same situation experienced by millions, the people who are physically active, avoid junk and fast foods, and try to eat "healthy whole grains."

Twenty years later, I exercise less intensively, don't restrict my fat, and eat NO "healthy whole grains" like those made of wheat. My HbA1c: 4.8%, fasting glucose 84 mg/dl—on no drugs. I am no longer diabetic.

Let the Wheat Lobby and its supporters march out the "whole grains have been proven to be healthier than white flour" argument. We all know that you cannot justify a food just because it is *less bad* than something else. *Less bad* does not necessarily mean *good*.

WEEK 8—DAY 1

DATE:	WEIGHT:
BLOOD PRESSURE:	BLOOD SUGAR A.M./P.M.: /

BREAKFAST:

SNACK 1:

LUNCH:

SNACK 2:

DINNER:

SNACK 3:

RATE QUALITY OF SLEEP:
(1 being the poorest and 5 being best)

| 1 | 2 | 3 | 4 | 5 |

RATE TODAY'S WHEAT TEMPTATION:
(5 being very strong cravings and 1 being no cravings at all)

| 1 | 2 | 3 | 4 | 5 |

RATE OVERALL MOOD:
(1 being the poorest and 5 being best)

| 1 | 2 | 3 | 4 | 5 |

ADDITIONAL COMMENTS/PROGRESS:

_____

_____

_____

_____

_____

_____

_____

_____

Reader Tip

"The important thing is to lose fat, and weight is not always the best way of evaluating that. I would encourage anyone who is discouraged about weight loss to take measurements and watch those numbers change, and not be so obsessed with the numbers on a scale."—Linda (Wheat Belly Blog reader)

WEEK 8—DAY 2

DATE:	WEIGHT:
BLOOD PRESSURE:	BLOOD SUGAR A.M./P.M.: /

BREAKFAST:

SNACK 1:

LUNCH:

SNACK 2:

DINNER:

SNACK 3:

RATE QUALITY OF SLEEP:
(1 being the poorest and 5 being best)

1   2   3   4   5

RATE TODAY'S WHEAT TEMPTATION:
(5 being very strong cravings and 1 being no cravings at all)

1   2   3   4   5

RATE OVERALL MOOD:
(1 being the poorest and 5 being best)

1   2   3   4   5

ADDITIONAL COMMENTS/PROGRESS:

_____

_____

_____

_____

_____

_____

_____

_____

_____

_____

_____

_____

_____

WEEK 8—DAY 3

DATE:	WEIGHT:
BLOOD PRESSURE:	BLOOD SUGAR A.M./P.M.: /

BREAKFAST:

SNACK 1:

LUNCH:

SNACK 2:

DINNER:

SNACK 3:

RATE QUALITY OF SLEEP:
(1 being the poorest and 5 being best)

| 1 | 2 | 3 | 4 | 5 |

RATE TODAY'S WHEAT TEMPTATION:
(5 being very strong cravings and 1 being no cravings at all)

| 1 | 2 | 3 | 4 | 5 |

RATE OVERALL MOOD:
(1 being the poorest and 5 being best)

| 1 | 2 | 3 | 4 | 5 |

ADDITIONAL COMMENTS/PROGRESS:

_____

_____

_____

_____

_____

_____

_____

_____

_____

_____

_____

_____

_____

WEEK 8—DAY 4

DATE:	WEIGHT:
BLOOD PRESSURE:	BLOOD SUGAR A.M./P.M.: /

BREAKFAST:

SNACK 1:

LUNCH:

SNACK 2:

DINNER:

SNACK 3:

RATE QUALITY OF SLEEP:
(1 being the poorest and 5 being best)

1	2	3	4	5

RATE TODAY'S WHEAT TEMPTATION:
(5 being very strong cravings and 1 being no cravings at all)

1	2	3	4	5

RATE OVERALL MOOD:
(1 being the poorest and 5 being best)

1	2	3	4	5

ADDITIONAL COMMENTS/PROGRESS:

_____

_____

_____

_____

_____

_____

_____

_____

_____

_____

_____

_____

_____

WEEK 8—DAY 5

DATE:	WEIGHT:
. BLOOD PRESSURE:	BLOOD SUGAR A.M./P.M.: /

BREAKFAST:

SNACK 1:

LUNCH:

SNACK 2:

DINNER:

SNACK 3:

RATE QUALITY OF SLEEP:
(1 being the poorest and 5 being best)

     1   2   3   4   5

RATE TODAY'S WHEAT TEMPTATION:
(5 being very strong cravings and 1 being no cravings at all)

     1   2   3   4   5

RATE OVERALL MOOD:
(1 being the poorest and 5 being best)

     1   2   3   4   5

ADDITIONAL COMMENTS/PROGRESS:

_____

_____

_____

_____

_____

_____

_____

_____

_____

_____

_____

_____

_____

_____

WEEK 8—DAY 6

DATE:	WEIGHT:
BLOOD PRESSURE:	BLOOD SUGAR A.M./P.M.: /

BREAKFAST:

SNACK 1:

LUNCH:

SNACK 2:

DINNER:

SNACK 3:

RATE QUALITY OF SLEEP:
(1 being the poorest and 5 being best)

1	2	3	4	5

RATE TODAY'S WHEAT TEMPTATION:
(5 being very strong cravings and 1 being no cravings at all)

1	2	3	4	5

RATE OVERALL MOOD:
(1 being the poorest and 5 being best)

1	2	3	4	5

ADDITIONAL COMMENTS/PROGRESS:

_____

_____

_____

_____

_____

_____

_____

_____

_____

_____

_____

_____

_____

WEEK 8—DAY 7

DATE:	WEIGHT:
BLOOD PRESSURE:	BLOOD SUGAR A.M./P.M.: /

BREAKFAST:

SNACK 1:

LUNCH:

SNACK 2:

DINNER:

SNACK 3:

RATE QUALITY OF SLEEP:
(1 being the poorest and 5 being best)

1   2   3   4   5

RATE TODAY'S WHEAT TEMPTATION:
(5 being very strong cravings and 1 being no cravings at all)

1   2   3   4   5

RATE OVERALL MOOD:
(1 being the poorest and 5 being best)

1   2   3   4   5

ADDITIONAL COMMENTS/PROGRESS:

_____

_____

_____

_____

_____

_____

_____

_____

_____

_____

_____

_____

Calories In . . . 8-Fold Calories Out?

The effect of wheat elimination on weight loss is intriguing.

I fully recognize that it defies credibility, but the typical effect of abrupt and total wheat elimination is weight loss of one pound per day. This translates to the equivalent of 3,500 calories (the calories contained in one pound of body fat) lost. How can this be? How can elimination of wheat—without limiting other calories, without cutting fat intake, without pushing the plate away or consuming smaller portions—lead to an incredible rate of weight loss equivalent to 3,500 calories lost per day? After all, elimination of wheat reduces calorie intake by 400 calories per day. That leaves 3,100 calories per day unaccounted for. Where do they go?

I don't have an answer . . . I can only speculate that, with elimination of wheat, the whole is greater than the sum of the parts, and 400 calories per day less consumed leads to the equivalent of 3,500 calories lost in weight because:

- Wheat elimination restores leptin sensitivity—*Resistance* to the hormone of satiety, leptin, leads to stalled weight loss efforts. The lectins in wheat have been shown, at least in an experimental animal model, to block the leptin receptor. Could it be that elimination of wheat restores leptin sensitivity? And does that somehow lead to accelerated metabolism?

- The weight lost is really water weight—I don't think this is likely to be entirely true, since there is such an large effect on reducing waist size. If you track waist circumference as you progress through your wheat-free experience, you will note substantial reductions in waist size. This is unlikely to represent water loss.

There is clearly something quite unique and not fully understood going on. I've seen it happen many, many times. Going wheat-free results in rapid weight loss at about the pound-a-day rate.

By the way, I'm starting to recognize the "experts" I'm debating on radio as those "educated" by the Wheat Trade Lobby when they say, "Calories in, calories out" and cutting wheat can only lead to weight loss in proportion to the calories reduced, wheat or otherwise. Their vigorous focus on this issue makes me believe that they, too, may know that there is potential for a unique weight-loss effect of wheat elimination but they deny it exists.

FAQ

What can you eat on a wheat-free diet?

Eat real, natural foods such as eggs, raw nuts, plenty of vegetables, and fish, fowl, and meats. Use healthy oils like olive, walnut, and coconut liberally. Eat occasional fruit and plenty of avocado and olives, and use herbs and spices freely. Eat raw or least cooked whenever possible and certainly do not frequent fast food places, processed snacks, or junk foods. While it may sound restrictive, a return to non-grain foods is incredibly rich and varied. Many people's eyes have been closed to the great variety of foods available to us minus the wheat.

WEEK 9—DAY 1

DATE:	WEIGHT:
BLOOD PRESSURE:	BLOOD SUGAR A.M./P.M.: /

BREAKFAST:

SNACK 1:

LUNCH:

SNACK 2:

DINNER:

SNACK 3:

RATE QUALITY OF SLEEP:
(1 being the poorest and 5 being best)

| 1 | 2 | 3 | 4 | 5 |

RATE TODAY'S WHEAT TEMPTATION:
(5 being very strong cravings and 1 being no cravings at all)

| 1 | 2 | 3 | 4 | 5 |

RATE OVERALL MOOD:
(1 being the poorest and 5 being best)

| 1 | 2 | 3 | 4 | 5 |

ADDITIONAL COMMENTS/PROGRESS:

_____

_____

_____

_____

_____

_____

_____

_____

Reader Testimonial

"After losing my 'wheat belly' I truly regained my youth! I am 69 years old and feel like I am in my 20s (energy, stamina). I am in great physical condition. I no longer need BP or triglyceride medication."—John (Wheat Belly Blog reader)

WEEK 9—DAY 2

DATE:	WEIGHT:
BLOOD PRESSURE:	BLOOD SUGAR A.M./P.M.: /

BREAKFAST:

SNACK 1:

LUNCH:

SNACK 2:

DINNER:

SNACK 3:

RATE QUALITY OF SLEEP:
(1 being the poorest and 5 being best)

1   2   3   4   5

RATE TODAY'S WHEAT TEMPTATION:
(5 being very strong cravings and 1 being no cravings at all)

1   2   3   4   5

RATE OVERALL MOOD:
(1 being the poorest and 5 being best)

1   2   3   4   5

ADDITIONAL COMMENTS/PROGRESS:

_____

_____

_____

_____

_____

_____

_____

_____

_____

_____

_____

_____

WEEK 9—DAY 3

DATE:	WEIGHT:
BLOOD PRESSURE:	BLOOD SUGAR A.M./P.M.: /

BREAKFAST:

SNACK 1:

LUNCH:

SNACK 2:

DINNER:

SNACK 3:

RATE QUALITY OF SLEEP:
(1 being the poorest and 5 being best)

1   2   3   4   5

RATE TODAY'S WHEAT TEMPTATION:
(5 being very strong cravings and 1 being no cravings at all)

1   2   3   4   5

RATE OVERALL MOOD:
(1 being the poorest and 5 being best)

1   2   3   4   5

ADDITIONAL COMMENTS/PROGRESS:

_____

_____

_____

_____

_____

_____

_____

_____

_____

_____

_____

_____

WEEK 9—DAY 4

DATE:	WEIGHT:
BLOOD PRESSURE:	BLOOD SUGAR A.M./P.M.: /

BREAKFAST:

SNACK 1:

LUNCH:

SNACK 2:

DINNER:

SNACK 3:

RATE QUALITY OF SLEEP:
(1 being the poorest and 5 being best)

| 1 | 2 | 3 | 4 | 5 |

RATE TODAY'S WHEAT TEMPTATION:
(5 being very strong cravings and 1 being no cravings at all)

| 1 | 2 | 3 | 4 | 5 |

RATE OVERALL MOOD:
(1 being the poorest and 5 being best)

| 1 | 2 | 3 | 4 | 5 |

ADDITIONAL COMMENTS/PROGRESS:

_____

_____

_____

_____

_____

_____

_____

_____

_____

_____

_____

_____

WEEK 9—DAY 5

DATE:	WEIGHT:
BLOOD PRESSURE:	BLOOD SUGAR A.M./P.M.: /

BREAKFAST:

SNACK 1:

LUNCH:

SNACK 2:

DINNER:

SNACK 3:

RATE QUALITY OF SLEEP:
(1 being the poorest and 5 being best)

| 1 | 2 | 3 | 4 | 5 |

RATE TODAY'S WHEAT TEMPTATION:
(5 being very strong cravings and 1 being no cravings at all)

| 1 | 2 | 3 | 4 | 5 |

RATE OVERALL MOOD:
(1 being the poorest and 5 being best)

| 1 | 2 | 3 | 4 | 5 |

ADDITIONAL COMMENTS/PROGRESS:

_____

_____

_____

_____

_____

_____

_____

_____

_____

_____

_____

_____

_____

WEEK 9—DAY 6

DATE:	WEIGHT:
BLOOD PRESSURE:	BLOOD SUGAR A.M./P.M.: /

BREAKFAST:

SNACK 1:

LUNCH:

SNACK 2:

DINNER:

SNACK 3:

RATE QUALITY OF SLEEP:
(1 being the poorest and 5 being best)

| 1 | 2 | 3 | 4 | 5 |

RATE TODAY'S WHEAT TEMPTATION:
(5 being very strong cravings and 1 being no cravings at all)

| 1 | 2 | 3 | 4 | 5 |

RATE OVERALL MOOD:
(1 being the poorest and 5 being best)

| 1 | 2 | 3 | 4 | 5 |

ADDITIONAL COMMENTS/PROGRESS:

WEEK 9—DAY 7

DATE:	WEIGHT:
BLOOD PRESSURE:	BLOOD SUGAR A.M./P.M.: /

BREAKFAST:

SNACK 1:

LUNCH:

SNACK 2:

DINNER:

SNACK 3:

RATE QUALITY OF SLEEP:
(1 being the poorest and 5 being best)

1	2	3	4	5

RATE TODAY'S WHEAT TEMPTATION:
(5 being very strong cravings and 1 being no cravings at all)

1	2	3	4	5

RATE OVERALL MOOD:
(1 being the poorest and 5 being best)

1	2	3	4	5

ADDITIONAL COMMENTS/PROGRESS:

_____

_____

_____

_____

_____

_____

_____

_____

_____

_____

_____

_____

_____

Gluten-Free Muffin Top

I know I've said this many times before, but it bears frequent repeating since so many people are waylaid by this "gluten-free" notion:

NOBODY should be eating gluten-free foods made with cornstarch, rice starch, tapioca starch, or potato starch. These starches in the dried, powdered form provide an exponential increase in surface area for digestion, thereby leading to sky-high blood sugar and all the consequences of extravagant glycation (glucose modification of proteins), such as diabetes, visceral fat accumulation, hypertension, cataracts, arthritis, low HDL/high triglycerides/increased small LDL particles, heart disease, and cancer.

In fact, one Wheat Belly Blog reader diagnosed with celiac disease was encouraged to try a gluten-free diet by her doctor. However, this diet resulted in dramatic weight gain and a muffin top, leaving the reader feeling very discouraged. But once she discovered the Wheat Belly diet and removed all grains from her diet, she began to lose her "wheat belly" within days.

So we don't replace one problem—modern semi-dwarf wheat—with another problem—gluten-free junk carbohydrates in this dried, pulverized form.

This is such an incredible blunder that is *growing* because, as more people embrace the idea of being gluten free, they turn to these foods that are now found in most grocery stores.

So let's be absolutely clear: Nobody should be eating these awful gluten-free foods made with junk carbohydrate ingredients! It may be "organic," "multigrain," "sprouted," "fair trade," or pink with purple polka dots . . . gluten-free foods made with cornstarch, rice starch, tapioca starch, and potato starch are unhealthy, and no one should eat them.

And, you know, it has often struck me as odd that some of the objections to the ideas brought forth in *Wheat Belly* come from the celiac and gluten-free communities. Take a look, however, at some of the gluten-free magazines, websites, and blogs and you will see prominent ads for gluten-free foods made with cornstarch, rice starch, tapioca starch, and potato starch.

FAQ

Will I be hungry on a wheat-free diet?

Recall that people who are wheat-free consume, on average, 400 calories less per day and are not driven by the 90-120 minute cycle of hunger that is common to wheat. It means you eat when you are hungry and you eat less. It means a breakfast of 3 eggs with green peppers and sundried tomatoes, olive oil, and mozzarella cheese for breakfast at 7 am and you're not hungry until 1 pm. That's an entirely different experience than the shredded wheat cereal in skim milk at 7 am, hungry for a snack at 9 am, hungry again at 11 am, counting the minutes until lunch. Eat lunch at noon, sleepy by 2 pm, etc. All of this goes away by banning wheat from the diet, provided the lost calories are replaced with real healthy foods.

WEEK 10—DAY 1

DATE:	WEIGHT:
BLOOD PRESSURE:	BLOOD SUGAR A.M./P.M.: /

BREAKFAST:

SNACK 1:

LUNCH:

SNACK 2:

DINNER:

SNACK 3:

RATE QUALITY OF SLEEP:
(1 being the poorest and 5 being best)

| 1 | 2 | 3 | 4 | 5 |

RATE TODAY'S WHEAT TEMPTATION:
(5 being very strong cravings and 1 being no cravings at all)

| 1 | 2 | 3 | 4 | 5 |

RATE OVERALL MOOD:
(1 being the poorest and 5 being best)

| 1 | 2 | 3 | 4 | 5 |

ADDITIONAL COMMENTS/PROGRESS:

_____

_____

_____

_____

_____

Reader Testimonial

"If stopping wheat had done nothing for me but get rid of the migraines, it would be worth it for that alone. But my chronic, annoying post-nasal drip and constant allergy symptoms have also disappeared; I've stopped needing a nap in the middle of the day; I've stopped having any food cravings. I have also been able to stop taking omeprazole for GERD—no digestion problems whatsoever now. My energy levels are much higher throughout the day, and a lot of small daily aches and pains—especially arthritis in my hands and fingers—have disappeared."—Lucas (Wheat Belly Blog reader)

WEEK 10—DAY 2

DATE:	WEIGHT:
BLOOD PRESSURE:	BLOOD SUGAR A.M./P.M.: /

BREAKFAST:

SNACK 1:

LUNCH:

SNACK 2:

DINNER:

SNACK 3:

RATE QUALITY OF SLEEP:
(1 being the poorest and 5 being best)

1   2   3   4   5

RATE TODAY'S WHEAT TEMPTATION:
(5 being very strong cravings and 1 being no cravings at all)

1   2   3   4   5

RATE OVERALL MOOD:
(1 being the poorest and 5 being best)

1   2   3   4   5

ADDITIONAL COMMENTS/PROGRESS:

_____

_____

_____

_____

_____

_____

_____

_____

_____

_____

_____

_____

WEEK 10—DAY 3

DATE:	WEIGHT:
BLOOD PRESSURE:	BLOOD SUGAR A.M./P.M.: /

BREAKFAST:

SNACK 1:

LUNCH:

SNACK 2:

DINNER:

SNACK 3:

RATE QUALITY OF SLEEP:
(1 being the poorest and 5 being best)

| 1 | 2 | 3 | 4 | 5 |

RATE TODAY'S WHEAT TEMPTATION:
(5 being very strong cravings and 1 being no cravings at all)

| 1 | 2 | 3 | 4 | 5 |

RATE OVERALL MOOD:
(1 being the poorest and 5 being best)

| 1 | 2 | 3 | 4 | 5 |

ADDITIONAL COMMENTS/PROGRESS:

_____

_____

_____

_____

_____

_____

_____

_____

_____

_____

_____

_____

_____

WEEK 10—DAY 4

DATE:	WEIGHT:
BLOOD PRESSURE:	BLOOD SUGAR A.M./P.M.: /

BREAKFAST:

SNACK 1:

LUNCH:

SNACK 2:

DINNER:

SNACK 3:

RATE QUALITY OF SLEEP:
(1 being the poorest and 5 being best)

1	2	3	4	5

RATE TODAY'S WHEAT TEMPTATION:
(5 being very strong cravings and 1 being no cravings at all)

1	2	3	4	5

RATE OVERALL MOOD:
(1 being the poorest and 5 being best)

1	2	3	4	5

ADDITIONAL COMMENTS/PROGRESS:

WEEK 10—DAY 5

DATE:	WEIGHT:
BLOOD PRESSURE:	BLOOD SUGAR A.M./P.M.: /

BREAKFAST:

SNACK 1:

LUNCH:

SNACK 2:

DINNER:

SNACK 3:

RATE QUALITY OF SLEEP:
(1 being the poorest and 5 being best)

| 1 | 2 | 3 | 4 | 5 |

RATE TODAY'S WHEAT TEMPTATION:
(5 being very strong cravings and 1 being no cravings at all)

| 1 | 2 | 3 | 4 | 5 |

RATE OVERALL MOOD:
(1 being the poorest and 5 being best)

| 1 | 2 | 3 | 4 | 5 |

ADDITIONAL COMMENTS/PROGRESS:

_____

_____

_____

_____

_____

_____

_____

_____

_____

_____

_____

_____

_____

WEEK 10—DAY 6

DATE:	WEIGHT:
BLOOD PRESSURE:	BLOOD SUGAR A.M./P.M.: /

BREAKFAST:

SNACK 1:

LUNCH:

SNACK 2:

DINNER:

SNACK 3:

RATE QUALITY OF SLEEP:
(1 being the poorest and 5 being best)

| 1 | 2 | 3 | 4 | 5 |

RATE TODAY'S WHEAT TEMPTATION:
(5 being very strong cravings and 1 being no cravings at all)

| 1 | 2 | 3 | 4 | 5 |

RATE OVERALL MOOD:
(1 being the poorest and 5 being best)

| 1 | 2 | 3 | 4 | 5 |

ADDITIONAL COMMENTS/PROGRESS:

_____

_____

_____

_____

_____

_____

_____

_____

_____

_____

_____

_____

_____

WEEK 10—DAY 7

DATE:	WEIGHT:
BLOOD PRESSURE:	BLOOD SUGAR A.M./P.M.: /

BREAKFAST:

SNACK 1:

LUNCH:

SNACK 2:

DINNER:

SNACK 3:

RATE QUALITY OF SLEEP:
(1 being the poorest and 5 being best)

1	2	3	4	5

RATE TODAY'S WHEAT TEMPTATION:
(5 being very strong cravings and 1 being no cravings at all)

1	2	3	4	5

RATE OVERALL MOOD:
(1 being the poorest and 5 being best)

1	2	3	4	5

ADDITIONAL COMMENTS/PROGRESS:

_____

_____

_____

_____

_____

_____

_____

_____

_____

_____

_____

_____

_____

Your Liver is Fat

A Wheat Belly Blog reader was once prescribed a low-fat diet after several tests that showed her having a fatty liver. This did not correspond with *Wheat Belly*'s suggestions to add healthy fats to daily eating, and the reader wondered how to reconcile the addition of healthy fats to her diet while also maintaining a low-fat regimen to please her doctor.

Does this sound familiar to you? If so, remember that it's not your job to please your doctor. It's your job to do *what's right for your health.*

A low-fat diet CAUSES fatty liver because cutting fat increases carbohydrate intake which, in turn, increases *de novo lipogenesis*, the conversion of carbohydrates to fats that are deposited in your liver.

In other words, feeding your liver more carbohydrates and less fat encourages the formation of triglycerides, some of which are released into the bloodstream as VLDL (very low-density lipoproteins), the rest of which remain in the liver. Triglycerides are fats, fats are triglycerides. As you eat more "healthy whole grains" and other foods that fit into a low-fat diet, your liver makes more triglycerides, your liver—along with your intestinal tract, pancreas, kidneys, and heart (percardial fat)—accumulates fat, gets larger, and increases markers of liver damage like AST and ALT. Over many years, this can lead to cirrhosis, identical to the disease generated by excessive alcohol consumption.

If dietary fat is made of triglycerides, doesn't this also cause fatty liver? No, because your liver's capacity to manufacture fats outweighs your ability to consume fat. Fats in the diet do indeed increase triglyceride levels in the blood . . . a little bit. But carbohydrates in the diet increase triglycerides . . . *a lot* (though the effect is delayed for several hours, sufficient to allow *de novo lipogenesis* to proceed).

Prescribing a low-fat diet is not only ineffective, but actually *causes* the problem it was meant to treat. This is like telling a smoker that they are short of breath because they don't smoke enough. Your liver is fat because you eat too much fat? Wow.

Any weight gain, acid reflux, or high blood pressure you may also suffer from is highly likely to be a consequence of our favorite carbohydrate to bash: wheat. Lose the wheat, lose the weight, lose the hypertension, lose the acid reflux . . . lose the fatty liver.

FAQ

So does going wheat free mean going gluten free?

Yes, but do *not* eat gluten-free foods! Let me explain.

Wheat raises blood sugar higher than nearly all other foods, including table sugar and many candy bars. The few foods that increase blood sugar *higher* than even wheat include figs, dates, and other dried fruits and rice starch, cornstarch, tapioca starch, and potato starch—the most common ingredients used in gluten-free foods. A gluten-free whole grain bread, for instance, is usually made with a combination of brown rice, potato, and tapioca starches. These dried pulverized starches are packed with highly digestible high-glycemic-index carbohydrates and thereby send blood sugar through the roof. This contributes to diabetes, cataracts, arthritis, heart disease, and growing belly fat. This is why many celiac patients who forgo wheat and resort to gluten-free foods become fat and diabetic. Gluten-free foods as they are currently manufactured are very poor substitutes for wheat flour.

Anyone who consumes gluten-free foods, like gluten-free muffins, should regard them as an occasional indulgence, no different than eating a bag of jelly beans.

WEEK 11—DAY 1

DATE:	WEIGHT:
BLOOD PRESSURE:	BLOOD SUGAR A.M./P.M.: /

BREAKFAST:

SNACK 1:

LUNCH:

SNACK 2:

DINNER:

SNACK 3:

RATE QUALITY OF SLEEP:
(1 being the poorest and 5 being best)

1	2	3	4	5

RATE TODAY'S WHEAT TEMPTATION:
(5 being very strong cravings and 1 being no cravings at all)

1	2	3	4	5

RATE OVERALL MOOD:
(1 being the poorest and 5 being best)

1	2	3	4	5

ADDITIONAL COMMENTS/PROGRESS:

_____

_____

_____

_____

_____

_____

Reader Tip

"Just reconnect with real food. Go back to the foods we've been told to avoid, like eggs, meats, and full-fat dairy. When you've mastered this big first step, then move on to the recipes that allow you to re-create pizza, chocolate chip cookies, and muffins—minus wheat, no gluten-free booby-trapped junk carbohydrates, no sugar—just delicious and healthy!"—Gary (Wheat Belly Blog reader)

WEEK 11—DAY 2

DATE:	WEIGHT:
BLOOD PRESSURE:	BLOOD SUGAR A.M./P.M.: /

BREAKFAST:

SNACK 1:

LUNCH:

SNACK 2:

DINNER:

SNACK 3:

RATE QUALITY OF SLEEP:
(1 being the poorest and 5 being best)

| 1 | 2 | 3 | 4 | 5 |

RATE TODAY'S WHEAT TEMPTATION:
(5 being very strong cravings and 1 being no cravings at all)

| 1 | 2 | 3 | 4 | 5 |

RATE OVERALL MOOD:
(1 being the poorest and 5 being best)

| 1 | 2 | 3 | 4 | 5 |

ADDITIONAL COMMENTS/PROGRESS:

WEEK 11—DAY 3

DATE:	WEIGHT:
BLOOD PRESSURE:	BLOOD SUGAR A.M./P.M.: /

BREAKFAST:

SNACK 1:

LUNCH:

SNACK 2:

DINNER:

SNACK 3:

RATE QUALITY OF SLEEP:
(1 being the poorest and 5 being best)

1	2	3	4	5

RATE TODAY'S WHEAT TEMPTATION:
(5 being very strong cravings and 1 being no cravings at all)

1	2	3	4	5

RATE OVERALL MOOD:
(1 being the poorest and 5 being best)

1	2	3	4	5

ADDITIONAL COMMENTS/PROGRESS:

_____

_____

_____

_____

_____

_____

_____

_____

_____

_____

_____

_____

WEEK 11—DAY 4

DATE:	WEIGHT:
BLOOD PRESSURE:	BLOOD SUGAR A.M./P.M.: /

BREAKFAST:

SNACK 1:

LUNCH:

SNACK 2:

DINNER:

SNACK 3:

RATE QUALITY OF SLEEP:
(1 being the poorest and 5 being best)

1	2	3	4	5

RATE TODAY'S WHEAT TEMPTATION:
(5 being very strong cravings and 1 being no cravings at all)

1	2	3	4	5

RATE OVERALL MOOD:
(1 being the poorest and 5 being best)

1	2	3	4	5

ADDITIONAL COMMENTS/PROGRESS:

_____

_____

_____

_____

_____

_____

_____

_____

_____

_____

_____

_____

_____

WEEK 11—DAY 5

DATE:	WEIGHT:
BLOOD PRESSURE:	BLOOD SUGAR A.M./P.M.: /

BREAKFAST:

SNACK 1:

LUNCH:

SNACK 2:

DINNER:

SNACK 3:

RATE QUALITY OF SLEEP:
(1 being the poorest and 5 being best)

1	2	3	4	5

RATE TODAY'S WHEAT TEMPTATION:
(5 being very strong cravings and 1 being no cravings at all)

1	2	3	4	5

RATE OVERALL MOOD:
(1 being the poorest and 5 being best)

1	2	3	4	5

ADDITIONAL COMMENTS/PROGRESS:

WEEK 11—DAY 6

DATE:	WEIGHT:
BLOOD PRESSURE:	BLOOD SUGAR A.M./P.M.: /

BREAKFAST:

SNACK 1:

LUNCH:

SNACK 2:

DINNER:

SNACK 3:

RATE QUALITY OF SLEEP:
(1 being the poorest and 5 being best)

| 1 | 2 | 3 | 4 | 5 |

RATE TODAY'S WHEAT TEMPTATION:
(5 being very strong cravings and 1 being no cravings at all)

| 1 | 2 | 3 | 4 | 5 |

RATE OVERALL MOOD:
(1 being the poorest and 5 being best)

| 1 | 2 | 3 | 4 | 5 |

ADDITIONAL COMMENTS/PROGRESS:

_____

_____

_____

_____

_____

_____

_____

_____

_____

_____

_____

_____

_____

WEEK 11—DAY 7

DATE:	WEIGHT:
BLOOD PRESSURE:	BLOOD SUGAR A.M./P.M.: /

BREAKFAST:

SNACK 1:

LUNCH:

SNACK 2:

DINNER:

SNACK 3:

RATE QUALITY OF SLEEP:
(1 being the poorest and 5 being best)

1	2	3	4	5

RATE TODAY'S WHEAT TEMPTATION:
(5 being very strong cravings and 1 being no cravings at all)

1	2	3	4	5

RATE OVERALL MOOD:
(1 being the poorest and 5 being best)

1	2	3	4	5

ADDITIONAL COMMENTS/PROGRESS:

Nails in the Coffin

There are several of what I call "nails in the coffin" for wheat. These are potential issues related to wheat that are *so* bad that, if any *one* of them proves true, then once and for all it will be goodbye to wheat's image as savior of health, protector of weight, darling of "official" agencies.

Among these nails in the coffin:

Gliadin as a cause of autism—We've all heard that autism has increased considerably over the past two decades, now affecting 1% of all children, and nobody knows why. Autistic kids have difficulty engaging in relationships and making friends with other kids, and usually have to be placed in special educational tracks to accommodate their unique needs.

Celiac disease can masquerade as autism, generating the full spectrum of the disorder. And mothers with rheumatoid arthritis and other autoimmune diseases and families with type 1 diabetes have increased likelihood of autistic children. We also know that autistic kids have an exaggerated reaction to wheat gliadin/gluten, along with increased likelihood of antibodies against gliadin. And wheat consumption has been associated with decreased fertility, suggesting an effect on the fetus and/or the uterine environment.

Can *in utero* exposure to wheat gliadin underlie the neurological changes that lead to autism in the newborn? If this relationship holds true, the lifelong implications for the child are so overwhelming that it can only mean that wheat has no role in the diet of any female contemplating pregnancy.

Wheat lectin as cause of leptin resistance—There is well-founded speculation that the lectin of wheat, *wheat germ agglutinin*, may be the instigator of *leptin resistance*. Leptin resistance is reflected by the paradoxic increase in leptin blood levels seen in overweight people. While increased leptin is supposed to *turn off* appetite and induce satiety, overweight and obese people have high levels of leptin *despite* their weight. This has been attributed to the condition of leptin resistance, the failure to respond to circulating leptin.

A group of investigators has speculated that lectins are perfectly crafted to be the trigger for leptin resistance. If true, it means that **Wheat Consumption = Weight Gain** via leptin resistance. It means that, in addition to the amylopectin A-induced straight-up rise in blood sugar/insulin and the appetite-stimulating effects of gliadin, wheat consumption = obesity.

Wheat lectins as a cause of gastrointestinal cancer—Could Steve Jobs, who died of pancreatic cancer, have actually died of long-term exposure to the lectins of wheat?

Think about it: People who eliminate wheat experience marked and often total relief from acid reflux, cramps and diarrhea of irritable bowel syndrome, improvement (and occasional cure) of ulcerative colitis and Crohn's disease. There are marked shifts in bowel bacteria and changes in pancreatic function with wheat elimination. If the irritative and inflammatory effects of wheat consumption on the gastrointestinal tract are so marked, and the effects of removal so dramatic, is it much of a leap to believe that the chronic inflammation and irritation caused by wheat could, over time, also lead to cancer?

After all, a major cause of cancer ("oncogenesis" or "tumorigenesis") is long-term, repetitive irritation and/or inflammation. The prolonged inflammation and irritation of ulcerative colitis, for instance, can result in colon cancer. People with celiac disease have increased risk for cancer of the small bowel, colon, biliary tract, and other gastrointestinal cancers. If we view celiac disease as just one end of the spectrum of wheat-related gastrointestinal irritation, then these conditions like acid reflux and irritable bowel syndrome that we might view as "celiac disease lite" may also heighten risk.

The Wheat Lobby and its friends in high places at the USDA, the U.S. Dept. of Health and Human Services, and other "official" providers of nutritional advice all agree: Replace white processed flour with whole grains, and incidence of cancer is reduced. While true, the effects of NO grains are what is in question.

Prediction: "Healthy whole grains" will prove to be the #1 most substantial cause, and thereby the #1 most preventable cause of gastrointestinal cancers.

Any one or all of these questions, if they hold true, will add a nail in the coffin for this incredibly corrupt invader of the human diet: "healthy whole grains."

WEEK 12—DAY 1

DATE:	WEIGHT:
BLOOD PRESSURE:	BLOOD SUGAR A.M./P.M.: /

BREAKFAST:

SNACK 1:

LUNCH:

SNACK 2:

DINNER:

SNACK 3:

RATE QUALITY OF SLEEP:
(1 being the poorest and 5 being best)

| 1 | 2 | 3 | 4 | 5 |

RATE TODAY'S WHEAT TEMPTATION:
(5 being very strong cravings and 1 being no cravings at all)

| 1 | 2 | 3 | 4 | 5 |

RATE OVERALL MOOD:
(1 being the poorest and 5 being best)

| 1 | 2 | 3 | 4 | 5 |

ADDITIONAL COMMENTS/PROGRESS:

_____

_____

_____

_____

_____

_____

_____

_____

_____

_____

Reader Testimonial

"I will never go back. I love what I eat now. My arthritis has diminished. I feel great."—Rick (Wheat Belly Blog reader)

WEEK 12—DAY 2

DATE:	WEIGHT:
BLOOD PRESSURE:	BLOOD SUGAR A.M./P.M.: /

BREAKFAST:

SNACK 1:

LUNCH:

SNACK 2:

DINNER:

SNACK 3:

RATE QUALITY OF SLEEP:
(1 being the poorest and 5 being best)

1	2	3	4	5

RATE TODAY'S WHEAT TEMPTATION:
(5 being very strong cravings and 1 being no cravings at all)

1	2	3	4	5

RATE OVERALL MOOD:
(1 being the poorest and 5 being best)

1	2	3	4	5

ADDITIONAL COMMENTS/PROGRESS:

_____

_____

_____

_____

_____

_____

_____

_____

_____

_____

_____

_____

_____

WEEK 12—DAY 3

DATE:	WEIGHT:
BLOOD PRESSURE:	BLOOD SUGAR A.M./P.M.: /

BREAKFAST:

SNACK 1:

LUNCH:

SNACK 2:

DINNER:

SNACK 3:

RATE QUALITY OF SLEEP:
(1 being the poorest and 5 being best)

1	2	3	4	5

RATE TODAY'S WHEAT TEMPTATION:
(5 being very strong cravings and 1 being no cravings at all)

1	2	3	4	5

RATE OVERALL MOOD:
(1 being the poorest and 5 being best)

1	2	3	4	5

ADDITIONAL COMMENTS/PROGRESS:

_____

_____

_____

_____

_____

_____

_____

_____

_____

_____

_____

_____

_____

WEEK 12—DAY 4

DATE:	WEIGHT:
BLOOD PRESSURE:	BLOOD SUGAR A.M./P.M.: /

BREAKFAST:

SNACK 1:

LUNCH:

SNACK 2:

DINNER:

SNACK 3:

RATE QUALITY OF SLEEP:
(1 being the poorest and 5 being best)

1	2	3	4	5

RATE TODAY'S WHEAT TEMPTATION:
(5 being very strong cravings and 1 being no cravings at all)

1	2	3	4	5

RATE OVERALL MOOD:
(1 being the poorest and 5 being best)

1	2	3	4	5

ADDITIONAL COMMENTS/PROGRESS:

WEEK 12—DAY 5

DATE:	WEIGHT:
BLOOD PRESSURE:	BLOOD SUGAR A.M./P.M.: /

BREAKFAST:

SNACK 1:

LUNCH:

SNACK 2:

DINNER:

SNACK 3:

RATE QUALITY OF SLEEP:
(1 being the poorest and 5 being best)

1	2	3	4	5

RATE TODAY'S WHEAT TEMPTATION:
(5 being very strong cravings and 1 being no cravings at all)

1	2	3	4	5

RATE OVERALL MOOD:
(1 being the poorest and 5 being best)

1	2	3	4	5

ADDITIONAL COMMENTS/PROGRESS:

_____

_____

_____

_____

_____

_____

_____

_____

_____

_____

_____

_____

_____

WEEK 12—DAY 6

DATE:	WEIGHT:
BLOOD PRESSURE:	BLOOD SUGAR A.M./P.M.: /

BREAKFAST:

SNACK 1:

LUNCH:

SNACK 2:

DINNER:

SNACK 3:

RATE QUALITY OF SLEEP:
(1 being the poorest and 5 being best)

1	2	3	4	5

RATE TODAY'S WHEAT TEMPTATION:
(5 being very strong cravings and 1 being no cravings at all)

1	2	3	4	5

RATE OVERALL MOOD:
(1 being the poorest and 5 being best)

1	2	3	4	5

ADDITIONAL COMMENTS/PROGRESS:

_____

_____

_____

_____

_____

_____

_____

_____

_____

_____

_____

_____

_____

_____

WEEK 12—DAY 7

DATE:	WEIGHT:
BLOOD PRESSURE:	BLOOD SUGAR A.M./P.M.: /

BREAKFAST:

SNACK 1:

LUNCH:

SNACK 2:

DINNER:

SNACK 3:

RATE QUALITY OF SLEEP:
(1 being the poorest and 5 being best)

| 1 | 2 | 3 | 4 | 5 |

RATE TODAY'S WHEAT TEMPTATION:
(5 being very strong cravings and 1 being no cravings at all)

| 1 | 2 | 3 | 4 | 5 |

RATE OVERALL MOOD:
(1 being the poorest and 5 being best)

| 1 | 2 | 3 | 4 | 5 |

ADDITIONAL COMMENTS/PROGRESS:

_____

_____

_____

_____

_____

_____

_____

_____

_____

_____

_____

_____

_____

Wheatlessness and the New "Normal"

Eliminate wheat from the diet and multiple facets of health improve. Health improves *so much* that I believe we have to reconsider what we regard as "normal"—normal health, normal aging, feeling good. If we accept the current state of the U.S. as it now stands, part of the current "normal" means being overweight or obese, being pre-diabetic, experiencing energy lows that impair day-to-day performance, developing arthritis by our 50s or 60s, osteoporosis, high cholesterol, hypertension, acid reflux, constipation, sleep disturbances . . . and on and on. These are the pedestrian plagues of the modern American, with a rare person who escapes all of it. Fiction imitates life, and we have become the Homer Simpsons of health: fat, lazy overeaters consigned to a life of discomfort, doctor visits, and prescription drugs. D'oh!

Taking wheat out of the health equation means that we need to *redefine* what we can expect in life. This is because eliminating wheat:

1. Reduces appetite—"Normal" calorie intake is, on average, 400 calories less per day for the wheatless. The notion that a 50-year-old, 150-pound woman needs 1,800 calories per day will need to be adjusted . . . downward.
2. Reduces body weight and visceral fat—You might need to shop in the junior dress sizes. Men may find that clothes manufacturers don't even make trousers for your waist size any more. (Ever try to find 31-inch waist pants?)
3. Reduces small LDL particles—Meaning risk for heart attack is dramatically reduced and the "need" for statin drugs is reduced or eliminated. It means that the fictitious target numbers your doctor treats known as "LDL cholesterol" will need to be readjusted to accommodate the *reduction*

or elimination of the true number one cause for heart disease in the U.S., small LDL particles.

4. Reduces blood sugar—Remove the amylopectin A of wheat and blood sugar drops, HbA1c (reflecting the previous 60-days blood sugar) drops, and resistance to insulin drops.

5. Diabetes and pre-diabetes are no longer inevitable—The CDC predicts that 1 in 3 Americans will be diabetic in the coming years, another 1 in 3 pre-diabetic—it is nearly everyone's fate, according to the numbers. Remove amylopectin A, remove lectin-induced leptin resistance, remove gliadin-induced appetite stimulation and diabetes and pre-diabetes for the most part *go away*.

6. Joint and bone health improve—Arthritis, joint pain, and osteoporosis, long considered the inevitable accompaniments of aging, are delayed or simply don't occur once the acidifying effects of wheat are removed, the inflammatory pus-like properties of visceral fat disappear, and brittle cartilage effects of amylopectin A–induced glycation no longer occur.

7. Glycation comes to a halt—Provided you don't feast on M&Ms and Coca-Cola in place of wheat, irreversible glucose modification of proteins—that causes hypertension, cataracts, osteoarthritis, left ventricular diastolic dysfunction (stiff heart), conduction system disease leading to heart rhythm disorders and pacemakers, nervous system impairment (reduced sensation and coordination), and aging—subsides to its natural slow level.

We also no longer need to resign ourselves to an inevitable future of drugs to deal with blood pressure, cholesterol, arthritis, acid reflux, and diabetes, along with "plenty of fiber" to compel our diseased colons to do their jobs. The savings in healthcare costs alone are mind-boggling.

Wheatlessness redefines what normal health and aging are all about. I predict that our perception that the "normal" 60-year-old, who is overweight and tired, who takes five prescription drugs, struggles to walk freely, and sees his or her doctor for multiple abnormal health conditions, will be replaced by a slender active person who can still run up a hill effortlessly, wear a bathing suit or bikini proudly at the beach, and sees a doctor for nothing more than a checkup.